Developmental Disorders of Language

Developmental Disorders of Language

Betty Byers Brown and Margaret Edwards

SINGULAR PUBLISHING GROUP, INC.
SAN DIEGO, CALIFORNIA

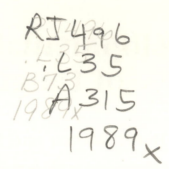

Phototypeset by Scribe Design, Gillingham, Kent
Printed in Great Britain by Athenaeum Press Ltd,
Newcastle upon Tyne

Introduction

We decided to write this book in the hope that we could bring together information and viewpoints from a number of sources, for the benefit of those who are about to enter the field of language disorders in a remedial capacity, or who may be returning to it, and for all those whose daily work brings them into close contact with children who have some language disability. The rapid growth of the subject and the variety of approaches it now encompasses, while making for a stimulating professional environment for those of us who are immersed in it, can be extremely confusing for those approaching it anew. It is very difficult to cover the current literature since it is generated by a number of different disciplines and therefore appears in a variety of professional publications. The student is forced to choose between what is topical and what is available. We hope that, at least, we can offer some guidance as to which aspects of the subject are current, which are evolving and which are of mainly historical interest.

We have, accordingly, adopted a liberal approach to the subject area. Since we wish to allow for changes taking place as knowledge accrues, we have tried to avoid adherence to any one theory or method. Nevertheless, we are aware that our selection of material will reflect our own interests and experience to a considerable extent. To select is to make some judgement as to what is important now and what is likely to become important in the future. We believe that early identification is vital to all therapeutic and educational approaches and we have therefore explored identification procedures in some detail. We further believe that effective therapy can only stem from sound hypotheses. We have therefore attempted to examine the theory behind the classification of language disorders and the evolution of clinical subtypes.

It is essential to offer some kind of unifying theory or model if a liberal approach is not to break down into unbridled eclecticism. We have chosen a language processing model because this seemed to be the best way of uniting order and flexibility. We have, however, tried to give prominence to the interactive aspects of language since we are convinced that language disorder cannot be viewed as a discrete condition associated with circumscribed pathology. In order to cover these topics, we have relied heavily on the work of others but inevitably we have shown bias in the selection of that work. There are still areas which we recognise as being important but which are not pursued in this text. There is no attempt to discuss language programmes, though we believe that their widespread use will demand a critical appraisal at some future date. Not, because of the rapid growth of research, have we considered the problems of older children or of those who acquire language disorder in early life as a result of trauma. The changing state of knowledge of these conditions will merit specialised publications. Throughout the text the close relationship which exists between written and spoken language disorder has been acknowledged by reference to the number of comprehensive publications which already exist in this field.

It will be apparent to the reader that we have drawn upon the ideas and findings of a large number of workers, many of whom are colleagues. Since the list would be too long for individual acknowledgement, we can only make this general statement of gratitude to all those who showed their generosity by sharing their research findings with us and by drawing our attention to other pertinent publications. We would also like to thank the reviewers who read the text before publication and who offered us perspicacious comments and thoroughly constructive criticism, together with encouragement.

We do, however, wish to acknowledge by name our colleague Catherine Duxbury who has assisted us in the preparation of this text. We are greatly beholden to her for prolific and punctilious reference work and for seeking out important papers which we might otherwise have missed. We are also extremely appreciative of the care she has shown in reading sections of the manuscript and in making detailed comments. The views of a representative of a new generation of research and clinical workers have been extremely valuable to us.

Finally, we offer this text in the hope that those entering the field of developmental language disorders will find in it the stimulation and satisfaction we have been fortunate enough to enjoy.

Betty Byers Brown
Margaret Edwards
March 1989

Contents

Chapter 1
Characterisation

Summary

This chapter describes those children who have developmental disorders of language and indicates how they may present to the lay public and to the professional. It discusses how the term 'developmental language disorder' has come to supersede earlier terminologies. Attention is drawn to the changes in thinking which the change in terminology represents. Estimates of prevalence, drawn from the literature of both speech impairment and language disability, are given. A theoretical framework is introduced within which language disorders in developing children may be considered. The pervasive nature of language disorder is emphasised together with its relationship to later learning disabilities. Illustrations are given as to how language disorder manifests itself at different stages of the child's development. This introduction paves the way for the specific processes of identification and management which are discussed in subsequent chapters.

Who are these children?

Children with developmental language disorders are those who are unable to communicate effectively through language or to use language as a basis for further learning. They are handicapped socially, educationally and, as a natural consequence, emotionally. Their handicap has been described as an invisible one because it is not obvious to the casual observer. There are no cosmetic or prosthetic signs to suggest that something is amiss. In the park, the playground or the shopping mall a language-disordered child may be indistinguishable from his normal peers. It is only the discerning observer or the professional who may see indications that the child is not fully equipped to take his place among his peers or that he is abnormally ill at ease in a social situation. Such indications include distress in a noisy or swiftly speaking environment; excessive restlessness or impulsivity;

immature and dependent behaviour; poor motor coordination; inappropriate speech or reluctance to make communicative contact, particularly with
strangers. These signs may alert the informed but will not carry the
message to the casual passer-by.

The lay person may first suspect that something is wrong when he or
she tries to engage the child in conversation or makes some overture to
which speech would be a natural response. The actual response may be
withdrawal or refusal, inappropriate clinging to the parent who may appear
over-protective or else a reply in speech which the person making the
overture may fail to understand. This person may react with affront or
embarassment and yet another situation has been created in which the
child feels inadequate and the parent ashamed or annoyed. The accumula-
tion of inadequacies as the result of these encounters may have a profound
effect upon the child's emotional well-being. If he is also being exposed
to continuous failure at school, the effect will be compounded. School
failure is difficult to avoid where there is language disorder because the
child is unable to master the structure of his native language or to use that
language creatively and flexibly. He may have reading and writing
difficulties in addition to his impaired oral communication. In view of the
heavy emphasis placed upon language in so many aspects of the school
curriculum and the fact that ability to comprehend language underpins so
many learning tasks, it will be difficult for a teacher to find a subject in
which the language-disordered child can excel.

The speech therapist in practice will encounter developmental language
disorder in all its manifestations at every stage of the child's development.
A very familiar introduction is through the child who presents with
delayed speech. A typical referral is that of a child, usually male, of between
2;6 and 3 years of age who uses a few words and no connected utterances.
Hearing tests reveal no impairment of acuity, psychological assessment
suggests that cognitive functioning is within normal limits. It will then fall
upon the speech therapist to establish whether or not the delay in speech
reflects a more serious disorder in the ability to acquire language. If so,
some indication must be given as to future educational needs in addition
to those of language therapy. The immediate course of action may involve
therapy for the child and guidance for the parents.

Alternatively, the young child may appear in the clinic with equivocal
responses to sound and speech and failure to comprehend spoken
language. Again, the course will be one of investigation and prediction
combined with immediate guidance and support. Other referrals may
include school-aged children who appear to be unable to organise their
spoken language in a coherent and fluent manner: those who are
experiencing reading difficulties which appear to be related to their
understanding and use of language, and children who have not eradicated
early speech problems which now appear to have another basis than

simple immaturity. These children will require full diagnostic linguistic assessment and a programme of remediation by therapist and teacher.

The speech therapist in training may encounter any of the cases mentioned above while carrying out practical work in a community clinic. Or, the first experience with developmental language disorders may be through visiting a language unit. In this case the student will look for some common denominator among the children. In a preschool unit this is likely to be delayed speech. It may be manifest in immature syntax, poor vocabulary or a restricted or unstable phonological system. The student may also be impressed by the children's low level of attention, particularly with regard to listening. Further observation may reveal a lack of symbolic play and deficiencies in behaviours such as turn-taking which normally precede communication through language.

If the first encounter with developmental language disorder comes about through visits to a regular primary or junior school for purposes of classroom observation, the child with a language disorder may appear to constitute a class of one. Beveridge and Conti-Ramsden writing for teachers (1987) give some indication of the range of behaviours which may be encountered: unintelligible speech; simple or limited expressive language; withdrawal and non-participation; inability to see a joke; literal mindedness; attention problems. It is only after considerable acquaintance with the process of language development that it is possible to begin to see how these behaviours may be united. The failure to master the basic underpinnings of language at an early age means that the skill may never be used with assurance and exactitude even though many of its components may eventually be mastered.

Byers Brown writing in an earlier publication [(Byers) Brown, 1971], pointed out the one characteristic that such children might have in common. Describing a group of language-disordered pupils gathered together for a summer school programme she observed 'They showed all kinds of learning and behaviour problems which seemed to stem from their disordered and confused speech' (p.85). With these problems were associated inattention, idiosyncratic spelling and poor physical coordination. 'The one thing that they had in common was an obvious and pervasive sense of failure.'

The sense of failure may be much less apparent once such children are placed in an educational environment where their needs are understood and the curriculum adapted to allow for full participation by all members of the class. Within a special school of this kind, the atmosphere will be buoyant and hopeful and the children lively and communicative. There are very few schools in the UK which cater specifically for the language disordered and these schools are highly selective as to which children they admit. They tend to receive those children with very severe disorders who cannot be managed within a local education system. Such children may have to be taught an alternative language system because spoken language may prove impracticable as a means of communication and systematic instruction. A person visiting such a school would receive a very different impression of 'language disorder' from that gained in any of the other situations described.

There are several professions which share responsibility for the care and management of language-disordered children but that of speech therapy demands the most continuous involvement. This is because so many disorders of language manifest themselves through delayed and disordered speech. It is also because the title 'speech therapist' in the UK carries the same connotation that 'speech–language pathologist' or 'language–speech therapist' does in other countries, namely involvement in all areas of language failure or breakdown. This responsibility means that language-disordered children place severe demands upon a speech therapy service. This is not due to sheer weight of numbers for, indeed, these have yet to be properly estimated. Rather it is due to the nature and course of language disorders which manifest themselves in many different ways and at different times. As a consequence, there is need for both flexibility and continuity in service provision and, where services are scantily funded and staffed, these requirements are difficult to meet and to maintain.

Table 1.1 shows in summary form some characteristic cases of language-disordered children as they present to the speech therapist.

Children with developmental disorders of language do not constitute the only group with difficulty in acquiring language. Among the others are those who suffer from hearing impairment, intellectual handicap or autism. Children who are socially disadvantaged may lack the opportunity to experience language in all its richness and so they may be slow to master it and use it with ease. Cerebral palsied children who are severely restricted in movement may be unable to experience the full range of language. They will be limited in their use of it as a tool even though they may be capable of mastering its basic structure. When there is more than one handicap, as in the case of a hearing-impaired child in an emotionally and socially impoverished home, the difficulties are, of course, compounded. In all these cases, the language handicap is secondary to another condition and would not have arisen in its absence.

What is a developmental language disorder?

The broad term 'developmental language disorder' simply denotes that something has gone wrong with the language behaviour of the developing child. It is a descriptive term which covers a range of conditions and impairments from word-finding difficulty to the inability to generate and maintain personal and social relationships through language. Bloom and Lahey in a text which has had a major influence upon the field (Bloom

Table 1.1 Characteristic cases of developmental language disorder

Age at referral (years)	Sex	Presenting symptom	History	Findings	Recommendations	Progress
2;6	M	Failure to produce words	Normal development apart from late sitting	Hearing and non-verbal intelligence normal; play limited and stereotyped	Language therapy and parent guidance	Very slow acquisition of all expressive language; problems persisting in articulatory precision
2;11	F	Failure to combine words	History unremarkable apart from head circumference in 90th percentile to height and weight in 50th percentile No neurological disorder	Hearing and cognitive development normal emotional maturity	Language monitoring and parent guidance	Steady growth in syntax and language use Phonology slow to develop but normal by 7 years
3;2	M	No sentences	Threatened abortion at 3 months but carried to term Born with cord around neck Late walking and clumsy; daytime enuresis, nail biting and hair pulling	Hearing within normal limits; wide scatter of ability shown on non-verbal intelligence; perceptuomotor problems	Language therapy	Language and learning difficulties persisting into junior school
2;6	M	No speech	Delivered by caesarean section because of placenta praevia Birthweight 9 lb 7 oz Milestones slightly delayed: sitting 10/12; walking 19/12	Responded to distraction testing at 40–60 dB	Further investigation and parent guidance Subsequent findings: suggested auditory processing difficulty and conductive loss Medical treatment improved hearing but poor auditory skills persisted	Persisting difficulty with comprehension and expression of language; word-finding difficulty

and Lahey, 1978) use the term as a descriptive label. They believed it to be necessary to use the term descriptively rather than diagnostically in order to refer to a range of behaviours without making a specific diagnosis on aetiological grounds or one which could imply permanent incapacity. As used currently, it covers all manner of deficits in oral comprehension and expression together with impairments of the written word.

As a generic class, developmental language disorder includes those few conditions which present as clearly definable and identifiable syndromes such as 'verbal auditory agnosia' (Rapin and Allen, 1983) and a much larger group of loosely classified behaviours such as 'language delay'. The term has emerged and established itself because of its clinical utility and its popularity is enhanced by its avoidance of controversial terminology. However, its use has done nothing to clarify the field which it represents. Schery (1985) reporting upon a recent and major investigation of language-disordered children found it necessary to qualify the label by adding 'labeled variously developmentally aphasic, dysphasic, language impaired, specific language disabled and language delayed'.

Developmental language disorder has no single aetiology. It exists with and without demonstrable neurological impairment. Whilst closely associated with hearing loss, intellectual handicap, emotional disturbance and environmental deprivation, it cannot be wholly explained by them since it is found in children who are normal in every other way. As has been stated, many conditions which reduce a child's capacity to move, reason and receive the normal range of experience also limit his language. However, the child with a language disorder shows perceptual and auditory inefficiency over and above any effects which could reasonably be expected from objective assessment of cognitive or hearing status (Eisenson, 1968).

Specific language disorder

The need to disassociate language disorders from other handicapping conditions and affirm them as handicapping in their own right has led to the use of 'specific' as a qualifier (Stark and Tallal, 1981; Gordon, 1987; Ripley, 1987). Whilst this places the emphasis firmly upon language as the source of the handicap, it tends to make for clumsiness without improving clarity. It is used by some for conditions where there is a proven neurological basis for the condition and by others for conditions defined by the exclusion of all other pathologies. Robinson (1987) uses the term with reference to a special school population with widely varying prenatal, postnatal and perinatal aetiologies. In a paper presented at the same time Snowling (1987) also uses the term 'specific' but applies it to 'language impairment' instead of 'language disorder'. Used with 'impairment' instead of 'disorder', the word 'specific' appears to have more exactitude, but we cannot assume that there is general agreement as to what constitutes this specific impairment.

To speak of language being disordered is to say nothing of the process which has brought it about. It is merely to give a name to a broad group of conditions which are related in so much as they affect language. It is useful to particularise the group even in such a broad way because it encourages us to examine the ways in which language that is disordered differs from language that is acquired in the normal manner and at a normal rate. It also prompts us to examine the ways in which language-disordered children differ from their normally developing peers without making aetiological assumptions. Nevertheless, it remains a broadly descriptive term to which the addition of the word 'specific' can only lend a spurious exactitude. It is quite possible that it is a term appropriate to this phase of our evolution of the subject which will be discarded when the conditions which it covers have been more clearly identified. We may see a return to a more specific terminology but one that is supported by the clear delineation of clinical subtypes. Alternatively, we may find that 'language disorder' has some utility when referring to a broad continuum within which certain conditions can be specified.

How prevalent is language disorder?

Present estimates of the prevalence of language disorder are likely to be less than accurate for the following reasons:

- The use of such terms as 'speech defect' and 'speech disorder' among early studies. These criteria have led to the acquisition of articulate speech being used as an outcome measure. As a consequence, the persistence of language difficulties has not been measured or represented.
- The inclusion of a number of known pathologies such as cerebral palsy, cleft palate and autism. These conditions are associated with difficulties and delays in acquiring speech and/or language but their inclusion prevents proper estimates as to the number of children whose handicap is restricted to the area of language.
- The lack of appropriate measures by which to assess both normal and deviant language development at the time when early surveys were undertaken.
- The differences in expertise and professional viewpoints of those taking part in the surveys.
- The lack of distinction between children with true language deficit and those with delays attendant upon socioeconomic status or cultural difference.

Unfortunately we cannot expect to gain a much clearer idea as to the numbers of children whose language abilities are impaired in relation to their other abilities until the field of language disorder is considerably clarified. The lack of conceptual clarity affects not only the way in which we treat these children but the way in which we identify and describe them. Berger (1987) points out that: 'epidemiological studies of particular forms of disorder cannot proceed until the phenomena of interest have been defined in ways that enable them to be discriminated and measured. These definitions then give rise to particular estimates of prevalence and incidence and can influence service provision and planning. Defined in other ways, different estimates may ensue.'

Nevertheless, in order to provide for language-disordered children in the immediate future, we have to make use of such figures as we have. Those surveys which are most frequently quoted will be presented and should be read with the above provisos in mind.

Surveys

A widely quoted survey is that undertaken by Morley and colleagues as part of a major study of 1000 families in Newcastle upon Tyne (Morley, Court and Miller, 1954; Spence *et al.*, 1954). The procedures and results as they pertain to speech development and disturbances and to early language development, are fully discussed by Morley in the original and revised texts of her classic work *The Development and Disorders of Speech in Childhood* (Morley, 1957, 1972). Morley reports a figure of 10% of children delayed in speech at 2 years of age, 6% at 3;9 and 3–5% at the time of school entry (4;9). She also records a figure of 3% with defects of speech and language at 6;6 years. Morley and her colleagues did not carry out detailed investigations into subsequent educational attainments so it is possible that some of her early speech delays did have persisting problems in associated areas of language. The fact that none of them was referred for special education is not necessarily significant.

MacKeith and Rutter (1972) in their note on the prevalence of speech and language disorders state that 1% of children come to school with a marked language handicap and that a further 4–5% may show sequelae of early language difficulties. A recent guideline from the Association For All Speech Impaired Children (AFASIC, 1988) states that the 1972 estimate is considered to be 'a gross underestimate and should be used as an indicator only'.

Marge, also reporting in 1972, indicated a 6.2% prevalence of language disability in pupils between the ages of 4 and 17 years in the US population. Tuomi and Ivanoff (1977) give an estimate of 6–7% for language disabilities among a kindergarten population and first grade population of 900 in Canada. This figure receives some support from a later Canadian study which finds 8.04% of 5-year-old kindergarten children showing language problems (Beitcham *et al.*, 1986).

Silva, in a recent publication (1987), reviews a number of epidemiological studies and points out that the more recent ones have tended to focus on the preschool child and particularly the 3 year old. He considers this to be because language develops dramatically in the preschool period. It could also be because investigators have more confidence in the measures which can be used at an early age because of our increased knowledge of early language development. If so, that confidence may be misplaced, certainly with regard to the stability of the findings. Many authors feel that it is not appropriate to use such terms as 'disability' or 'disorder' about the language of very young children since delay in acquisition may prove to be transient. Estimates of language delay in preschool children do not necessarily distinguish between levels of delay. The following studies are those in which some distinctions are made.

Stevenson and Richman (1976) identified 3–4% of 705 3-year-old children as language delayed by at least 6 months. Fifty per cent of the children so delayed were generally retarded. Only four children had roughly normal cognitive ability in conjunction with significant language delay. Randall, Reynell and Curwen (1974) in a study of 300 3 year olds found only one case of a specific, significant language delay which was still present at 4 years. The authors discuss this finding in relation to the prevalence figure of 1% yielded by other studies (Herbert and Wedell, 1970; MacKeith and Rutter, 1972) and to the estimate range of 1–0.7% per 1000. They conclude that 'if, as seems likely, a true developmental language disorder occurs to approximately the same extent as other developmental disorders (i.e. not more than 1 to 2 per 1000)' (p. 15) then their sample which was reduced by attrition to 160 'was much too small'.

Fundudis, Kolvin and Garside (1979) found that, of 3300 Newcastle children, 4% were speech retarded in that they were not using words strung together to make sentences. This 4% was considered to be a conservative estimate. Their follow-up procedures revealed that 18 of the children could be classified under 'pathologically deviant'. One of these was classified as 'severe dysphasia' but the others were in non-linguistic pathological categories. The remaining 84 children were classified as having a 'residual speech handicap' and their prevalence estimate was about 2–3% of children of school age.

Silva (1980) reporting on his sample of 937 3-year-old children in New Zealand gave a figure of 8% as being significantly delayed in either language expression (2%), language comprehension (3%) or both (3%). The most stable figure was that given for both comprehension and expression and this included a high percentage of children who were intellectually retarded or borderline.

In one of the few studies of 2 year olds, Rescorla (1984) gives an estimate of 10% language delay. She explains the discrepancy between this figure and the percentage generally estimated for 3 year olds (3–5%) by suggesting that some percentage of 2 year olds will surely have developed normal speech by three. Rescorla's figure is based upon a sample of 351 children between the ages of 22 and 26 months. There is good agreement between her figures and Morley's early findings on delayed speech development, with the same argument of delayed maturation advanced by both. The first findings of a collaborative study in the US (Kagan, unpublished paper, 1988) give a prevalence estimate of 8% in children of 1–3 years of age. These children failed a screening test standardised for their age group (Coplan, 1983). Serious delay in expressive language was found to be more frequent than in receptive language, 40% as against 27%. We have, as yet, no way of knowing whether these earlier signs will be upheld by subsequent findings, or whether they represent transient delays.

The most recent report received, that of the Invalid Children's Aid Nationwide (ICAN, 1988) accepts a figure of 0.08 as the prevalence for 'specific language disorders' and points out that the prevalence of language disorders among the preschool population is greater than for the school-aged population. This report makes clear distinction between language delay and language disorder. The bulk of the report is devoted to provision for school-aged children. Extrapolating from the findings of the 1972 paper (MacKeith and Rutter, 1972) the authors estimate that the current UK population of school-aged children will contain approximately 5600 who are language disordered. They estimate that as 'it is generally accepted that the prevalence of language handicap decreases with age' (p. 4) more than half of the children will be between the ages of 5 and 11.

We have no clear estimates of numbers of children who show reading or writing disorders later in school life as a symptom of continuing language disorder. However, the association between early language delay and disorder and subsequent learning disability is very strong (Strominger and Bashir, 1977; Aram and Nation, 1980; Silva, McGee and Williams, 1983; Snowling, 1987; Tallal, 1987). We may expect to gain more information in the future through the longitudinal studies now in progress (Bishop and Edmundson, 1987a; Tallal and Curtiss, cited in Tallal, 1987). It is therefore possible that the 1% estimate will be revised. Even if it is not, this cold little statistic still represents a great deal in terms of human misery and wasted potential. Those in the remedial professions will find in it evidence enough to continue to revise and extend their skills on behalf of the language disordered.

Speech therapists may deduce from such figures as we have, that they will have a responsibility towards all school-aged children with disordered language which will occupy a considerable amount of corporate clinical time. It will almost certainly be exceeded by their involvement with preschool children. They will be required to participate in investigations aimed at clarifying which delays are transient and which are associated with continuing disorders. They will be involved in programmes of guidance and prophylaxis and in individual therapy. Whatever the exact figures on language delay, it is continuously cited as the most common developmental problem found in preschool children (Bax, Hart and Jenkins, 1980; Snyder-McClean and McClean, 1987). The trend toward early investigation and intervention is extremely marked in the UK, the USA, Canada, Australia and New Zealand and is likely to continue.

How long have we known about language disorder?

One predictable consequence of a changing terminology is that it tends to suggest that a new group of children has been discovered. In some instances this is justified but the case of 'developmental language disorders' is not one of them. The children have been discussed and described for many years but under a number of different labels. A new label shows either an increase in knowledge or a change in thinking or both. It should not prevent students and clinicians from studying cases labelled by other names or texts using different terminology. To do this would be to negate a great deal of professional knowledge. The following historical review will draw attention to the change in terminology and indicate how it reflects changes in thinking.

Developmental aphasia

The term 'developmental aphasia' may be found in the literature of language pathology from its inception and is well represented in the period from 1950 to 1970. The last text published in the UK under the name developmental dysphasia was that edited by Wyke in 1978. This text contains valuable and pertinent information for all those concerned with developmental language disorders. Chiat and Hirson, in a much more recent publication (1987), select the term 'dysphasia' as being the most appropriate for the case under discussion. The term is obviously too useful to die away and is likely to be brought back into use for a specific category of language disorder (see also Heywood and Canavan, 1987). The move away from general use was part of the reconsideration of the receptive–expressive dichotomy which dominated the clinical language field and which owed its origins to the study of acquired aphasia in adults. Terminology based upon the receptive–expressive language model was current at the time when British speech therapists were starting to publish their findings. These added considerably to the sparse publications of the few neurologists and paediatricians who were interested in speech and language disorders. Conspicuous among speech therapists was the work of Morley (Morley *et al.*, 1954; Morley, 1957, 1960). Morley contributed a number of case studies on developmental aphasia and discussed how the condition might be differentiated from delayed speech. Cases of both receptive aphasia (with and without hearing loss) and expressive aphasia are cited. Expressive aphasia is illustrated in cases with and without cerebral palsy. Developmental aphasia is associated in all cases with neurological dysfunction but described in terms of delayed neurological maturation for the central processes involved.

Griffiths (1964, 1972) describes and discusses cases of both receptive and expressive developmental aphasia drawn from the records of the John Horniman School. This establishment, like its sister school, Moor House, was strongly influenced in its diagnostic determinations by the work of the medical director Worster-Drought. Worster-Drought's name is strongly associated with the condition of 'congenital auditory imperception' which he first identified. This condition is closely allied to Rapin's more recent 'verbal auditory agnosia'. The inability of some children to recognise the meaning of speech sounds which both these terms represent, is continuously documented in the literature of both hearing and language disorders (Ingram, 1959; McGinnis, 1963; Worster-Drought, 1965; Taylor, 1966; Morley, 1973; Ward and McCartney, 1978). The influence of Worster-Drought is recognised by a number of authors in the 1960s (Lea, 1965; Gordon, 1966; Thomas, 1969) including teachers, therapists and neurologists. Lea was one of the many workers at that time who also emphasised the symbolic nature of the aphasic disturbance in receptive aphasia.

The paediatric neurologist, Ingram, writing in 1965, also discusses receptive, developmental aphasia using it synonymously with 'congenital auditory imperception,' 'central deafness' and 'developmental auditory dysfunction'. The aphasias appear in the language branch of his classification of specific speech disorders, a process which would certainly be reversed in current classifications. Ingram describes the condition of receptive aphasia as 'immature patterns of speech–sound production and immature patterns of spoken language with difficulty in comprehending speech (sometimes with seeming sensory deafness)' (p. 5). Like other authorities (Gordon, 1966; Petrie, 1975) Ingram gives a poor prognosis for children with receptive aphasia believing them likely to be continuously and severely handicapped in educational attainment. He gives a better prognosis for the expressive category which comprises 'immature patterns of speech–sound production and immature patterns of spoken language' (p. 5). He states that the majority of children in this group will attain normal speech by 7 years of age. Ingram does not indicate whether or not these children will be free of subsequent learning difficulties, though he does say that children with retarded speech development have greater difficulty in learning to read and write than do normal children.

Greene (1964) points out some of the ambiguities inherent in the term 'aphasia' as applied to developmental states. Many speech therapists considered that there was sufficient similarity between the developmental and acquired adult condition for the same term to be used. This view was opposed by the neurologists. Some investigators therefore restricted their use of aphasia in childhood to the acquired state. Greene states that the term should never be used for delays in speech and language which are transcended by 5 or 6 years of age. However, she later indicated that there was no way of knowing which delays would recover by that time and which would not. One must deduce that the term 'aphasia' was not to be used until around 6 years of age when the delays were characterised as gross and persisting and carried a poor prognosis.

In the same paper (1964) Greene refers to the incomplete nature of investigations carried out into developmental aphasia, much of which she attributes to specialist bias. Representatives of different professions would look only for those signs which they perceived as significant. A notable example was that of the neurologists who would not take language delays seriously in the absence of clear or 'hard' neurological signs. Since the medical profession carried major responsibility for referring children for therapy and special education, this attitude was a source of considerable frustration to therapists and teachers as well as to parents. Although medical literature distinguished between 'developmental aphasia' and transient speech delays there was no correspondence between the developmental aphasia group and those few children who showed sufficiently clear signs of neuropathology to satisfy the neurologists. The term 'developmental aphasia' seemed thus to invite controversy while not assisting remediation. It is not surprising that workers in the field became dissatisfied with it. Greene points out that many authorities preferred to use a term which could cover the range of speech delays and yet could also be used to refer to the severe and prolonged state of developmental aphasia. Developmental language disorder accordingly started to replace 'developmental aphasia'.

The term 'language disorders' gained rapid popularity in the USA under such notable championship as that of Berry (1969). Berry propounds a concept of language behaviour which involves psychoneurology, psycholinguistics and psychophysiology and states that equipped with this knowledge 'the student should be ready to tackle the diagnostic study and teaching of children who find language learning difficult'. She emphasises the rigour of the undertaking and, indeed, it does take all her bright images to make it attractive. Fortunately, an alternative is offered. 'The student will find greater profit in studying the profiles of children who are handicapped by disabilities in language than by discursive chapters on symptoms and aetiology' (1969, p. 4). The emphasis on language profiles as a valuable way of understanding language disorders, has been a continuing feature for the last 20 years. All texts on the subject make use of a variety of case histories to indicate the range, diversity and also the common features of the condition. Table 1.2 shows profiles of two children with the terminology common to the 1960s and to the present day.

These two profiles have been selected from the literature because they deal with very different children. There can therefore be no attempt to make direct comparison between them in order to suggest the improvement of one kind of terminology over another. The case described by

Table 1.2 Changes in terminology for assessment and classification

*Assessment of Julie in 1964**		*Assessment of Tony in 1986†*	
Age at assessment (years)	4; 7	Age at assessment (years)	3; 4
Developmental history	Pneumonia at 9 months with anoxia and loss of consciousness Delayed milestones: walked at 18 months	Developmental history	General development normal Excellent self-help skills Early communication development normal Stopped communicating and responding to language in second year
Speech development	No babbling First words at 4 years Some difficulty with chewing and swallowing	Hearing	Within normal limits
Merrill–Palmer Scale	CA 4;6 MA 5;1	Assessment through observation	The following functions were described over time: pragmatic verbal comprehension syntax and phonology non-verbal abilities
Speech assessment	Could imitate individual consonants but had difficulty organising phonemic sequences No dyspraxia Poor auditory retention Unable to imitate even a simple rhythm No hearing loss Good auditory discrimination	Progress	There is progression from purely imitative responses to appropriate responses although some language forms presented difficulty Spontaneous conversation initiated at 5;4 years
		Standardized tests of language	Scored very poorly at 4 years RDLS CA 6;11 Age level 4;11 PLS CA 6;11 Age equiv. 6;6
Subsequent assessment measures:	Terman–Merrill IQ 91 WISC CA 8;6 Verbal scale 86 Performance 93 Peabody CA 8;6 Peabody MA 6;1 Bender–Gestalt Performed poorly	Cognition	Consistently scored above average on Leiter International Performance Scale However, appeared to have specific non-verbal difficulties in areas of verbal reasoning distinguishing between essential/accidental information and developing generalised flexible scripts
Diagnosis	*Developmental aphasia* Difficulties in auditory recall and comprehension of abstract speech; impaired syntax and grammar	Diagnosis	*Semantic–pragmatic language disorder* Conversational disability

*From Greene (1964).
†From Conti-Ramsden and Gunn (1986).

Greene could be assessed and described today with only slight differences in terminology and an extended range of procedures. The case presented by Conti-Ramsden and Gunn would not have been described earlier within the language impairment category since speech therapists lacked the techniques and concepts to work with such children. Both cases (Greene, 1964; Conti-Ramsden and Gunn, 1986) should be read in full for the issues they raise and the insights they reveal.

A theoretical framework

Reliance upon case history study alone is unwise since no student can hope to encounter the whole range of language disorders thereby. It is necessary to have some kind of theoretical framework within which each individual aspect can be placed. It is unlikely that specialist bias can be eliminated, even in the construction of such frameworks. Scholars and clinicians will approach the subject through the portal most accessible to them. They will tend toward approaches with which they are professionally most comfortable because most familiar. It is not desirable that specialist bias be eliminated altogether since it also brings specialist insight. However, it must be controlled and subjected to multidisciplinary discussion and appraisal. Medically based hypotheses involving genetic or neuropathological aetiologies will be of most service when tested against a number of other causal correlates. It may fall to the psychologist to generate a model which accounts for all the variables and allows them to be tested. The therapist and teacher will share the interest in constructing and testing such models. However, their overriding concern is to provide remedy. Consequently the search for a common cause may be of less interest than the search for a method which will allow many language-disordered children to be helped. Any method which seems to promise such help can then be tested in the proving ground of clinic or classroom. We are well past the point where any apology need be made for such an approach. The feedback of observation and deduction from children's response to treatment may be of vital importance in establishing the nature of the problem.

The nature of unifying hypotheses and causal correlates will be discussed further in Chapter 2 (Identification) because they profoundly affect identification procedures. It is difficult to handle all the possibilities without some concept of how language is processed by the brain. The move away from looking at language disorders as a number of discrete entities makes it necessary to postulate a framework within which they can be seen as points on a continuum. The continuum will cover factors within the individual's ability to process language and those outside or environmental factors which impinge upon this processing. Thus, a breakdown in language processing will cause a more or less severe disorder according to the effect of environmental factors. The severity of the disorder will also depend upon the profundity of the breakdown and the number of processes which are involved. Models of language processing will be discussed more fully in Chapter 4. They are also explored in a number of other texts, an excellent discussion being offered by Butler (1984). They arise from theories of information processing as these can be focused upon language. Even a simple model of language processing must include the following stages:

1. Communicative intent and content to be communicated.
2. A framework through which expression can be made.
3. Assembly of a motor programme to execute the communication.
4. Execution of the programme through organised sequences of neuro-muscular actions.

To these bare bones must be added word retrieval mechanisms, the ability to feed information forward and back and the facility for modifying the performance on receipt of feedback. This covers only part of the processing. If language is to be comprehended and acted upon there must be:

5. Signal detection or awareness of stimulus.
6. Attention to the stimulus also involving rejection of accompanying noise.
7. Recognition.
8. Memory.
9. Synthesis of all the above in order to build up a composite of all the information.

It is not difficult to consider such a model as it can be applied to the perfected skill. An adult well versed in communication makes use of all the above and has the ability to reflect upon his performance. Thus not only language but metalanguage is involved. When the model is applied to the developmental skill it becomes more difficult to sort out what is going on. Berger (1987) points out the difficulty of translating phenomena associated with the mature state to 'the realm of emerging forms and indefinite boundaries'. Present considerations of development have come about since many of our ideas on language have settled into precept and reappraisal is not easy. Some application can be made in that we may be able to identify points of breakdown or difficulty in the child's emerging skill. What is more taxing is to sort out the time when this difficulty heralds a permanent handicap or the point at which the child is unable to compensate by means of his other abilities.

Children who are developing language are also developing strategies through which that language can best be handled. In the case of language disorder, the child may either be unable to develop such strategies or may develop strategies which are not very efficient. Sometimes they are efficient for the one purpose but restrict subsequent language growth. The following illustration may be helpful here.

> S. aged 4;10 was referred to the Speech and Hearing Clinic by his primary school teacher because of 'unclear speech' and attention problems. The case history was one of delayed speech development with slowness in combining words and poor intelligibility. While his parents had noted these things, they had attributed them to general delay consequent upon poor health in infancy. S. was born with a heart defect which was corrected by surgery in his third year of life. S's mother had expected the speech difficulty to resolve itself 'especially when he got to school'. She had noticed that S. had poor attention but thought of this as an irritating piece of behaviour in an otherwise happy and compliant child. She considered that he might have been indulged a little because of his heart condition and, again, expected school to accelerate the process of maturity and control.
>
> Upon examination, S. proved to have normal auditory acuity but poor listening skills. He had difficulty with sound discrimination and in responding to a series of instructions. Comprehension was markedly impaired and this reduced his performance not only in language tasks but in cognitive ones. S.'s poor listening skills appeared to be the main factor in his reduced intelligibility since motor control and speech—sound production were within normal limits. The following behaviour was characteristic.
>
> > Clinician: 'What's the boy doing?'
> > S.: 'What boy doing?'
> > Clinician: 'You tell me. What's the boy doing?'
> > S.: 'What boy doing?'

It appears that S. is unable to interpret the 'what' question and repeats it, either to gain more information or to disguise his lack of understanding. It would be important for therapy to establish which strategy he is using. His repeated response to 'You tell me' could also be interpreted as failure to understand the real content of the request. He might have thought that 'You tell me' meant that he was to tell or repeat 'What is the boy doing'. An older child might clarify by asking 'What do you want me to say?'. Young children and language-disordered children will not do this because they lack the pragmatic skills to reach below the surface words and respond to the intention of the speaker.

When S.'s behaviour is seen in relation to the simple processing model he shows breakdown at stages (6), (7) and (9). His immature syntax suggests that there is some effect upon stage (2) and certainly upon overall monitoring of his own performance. An investigation at a much younger age would probably have shown first difficulties at stage (1). Seen as one condition within a broad spectrum of language disability, S. is placed toward the mild end of the spectrum within the group characterised by comprehension deficit. The impact of his environment cannot be fully assessed in retrospect. Its supportive elements have allowed him to continue to relate and to communicate without withdrawal or severe behaviour problems. He has developed some communicative strategies which are not particularly efficient but they serve to keep the interaction going and to allow the child more time to process the message. In a harsher environment, S. might have become much more distressed and withdrawn. Had attention not been focused upon his early health, his abnormal responses to sound might have prompted earlier referral. On the other hand, it is reasonable to look for some association between his heart condition and his other developmental difficulties.

The therapist would want to intervene in order to strengthen S.'s whole language matrix. Special attention would be paid to the improvement of listening and to teaching word meaning. The combination of these two skills should improve comprehension. The therapist would then demand a higher standard of word monitoring and might also attempt to teach the child other ways of clarifying meaning, e.g. 'Tell me again' 'Say it slowly' and eventually 'I don't understand'. A major responsibility would be to cooperate with teacher and psychologist in developing a suitable reading and writing programme. A further responsibility would be to explore the role of language in the school curriculum and attempt to estimate the support that S. would need in the future. As a child works his way through primary to secondary school, the language demands increase and these must be anticipated by the remedial service. Seen in reference to the language processing model, S.'s problem may be shown to affect all language skills since it constitutes a failure to perceive the nature of words. Both word boundaries and word meanings will suffer.

Continuum of disability

Reference has already been made to a continuum of language disability. This implies that a language problem will continue to spread. It is the pervasion of a number of skills that makes the condition impossible to treat on a once-and-for-all basis. In 1977 Strominger and Bashir presented a study based upon clinical records of language-disordered children first seen in the clinic at under 5 years of age and subsequently seen between the ages of 9 and 11. They reported that no child was entirely free from residual deficits. Examination of a number of aspects of language and learning showed a wide range of abnormality. The authors suggested that children who failed to acquire oral language would have difficulty in the acquisition of all language systems because of general problems posed by the grammar and its representation, regardless of form. Only 5% of the children in their sample had reading skills appropriate for their age. None of the children had been diagnosed as mentally handicapped and their educational failure was thus specifically linked to their language failure.

Byers Brown and Beveridge (1979) in an introduction to a workshop for teachers posed a number of questions representing queries which have recurred throughout the history of language disorders.

- Is there a continuum of language disturbances seen initially in the acquisition of the spoken word and later revealed as deficits in the secondary systems of reading and writing?
- Can we assume that all children with initial disorders of language must be at risk educationally?
- Is there one underlying factor which is causal and thereby links all language manifestations? Or, are the skills all related by factors in the child's disposition, neurological, emotional or environmental but not causally linked?
- Are different language and learning problems occurring independently in vulnerable children rather than being bound together by one definable disability?

Most authorities incline to answer 'yes' to the first question (Aram and Nation, 1980; Wiig and Semel, 1980; King, Jones and Lasky, 1982; Cooper, 1985). The answer to the second question is almost certainly 'yes' if we can also assume that the initial disorders were correctly diagnosed as affecting language and not articulation of speech. Where the child presents with initial problems of speech production only, pervasive language difficulty with its implications for education is not the likely outcome. However, articulation difficulties have been shown to be associated with reading problems. Where these reading problems do occur, they have a better prognosis than the difficulties associated with language impairment (Hall and Tomblin, 1978; King, Jones and Lasky, 1982). Children presenting with delayed speech will be found to be at educational risk when the delay is the outcome of difficulty in synthesising a number of language processes, or when the delay stems from or leads to severe emotional disorder. If the speech delay is the result of hearing or intellectual impairment the child will be at risk educationally because of his primary impairment.

The answers to the next two questions are not readily available and the considerations which they require will be pursued in Chapters 2 and 7. Since Chapter 2 deals with identification, it will discuss those populations within which the language disordered are most likely to be found as well as discussing their identifying signs. The discussion of clinical subtypes in Chapter 7 will consider how relationships between certain behaviour may be traced. The nature of the continuum model will be further discussed in Chapter 6 (The nature of language disorders).

In view of the complexity and diversity of the conditions grouped together under the broad heading of 'language disorder', it is not surprising to find that there were some reservations to the use of the term when first propounded on the grounds that it suggested a homogeneity which was not there to be found. Not only do the children in the group show different symptoms from each other but they have entered the group by different routes. Some are positively diagnosed as having a language disorder on the basis of tests constructed for the purpose. Others have been identified by exclusion: the child is not deaf, not intellectually retarded in the general sense, not autistic, not dysarthric and so must be language disordered. Had we arrived at more positive forms of identification at a point coincident with our developing interest (i.e. in the 1960s and 1970s), the subsequent paths of both children and professionals would have been a great deal easier.

Bases for differentiation

The process of differentiating language disorders has comprised the following approaches:

- Attempts to differentiate between abnormal language behaviour, which signified other handicapping conditions, notably hearing loss and cognitive impairment, and that which was rooted in language itself.
- Attempts to differentiate between the rate and manner in which language is normally acquired in infancy and abnormalities in this acquisition.
- Attempts to differentiate between individual language disorders or groups of disorders.

Handicapping conditions

The aim of differentiations such as those listed above was, and is, to provide appropriate help. It is important to make clear that differentiation does not mean segregation. At the present time the prevailing philosophy is one of integrated education for handicapped and normally developing children. We do not wish to categorise children in order to put them apart but in order to find ways of allowing them to enter into the community. If a child is wrongly diagnosed as hearing impaired and given a hearing aid when acuity is normal, that child cannot be expected to improve. The question of whether placement should be in a special school for hearing-impaired children or in mainstream school with hearing aid and other support does not arise. The child will benefit from neither.

The emergence of children who appeared to be deaf but failed to respond to methods of education designed for deaf or hearing-impaired children, led such pioneers as McGinnis in the USA and the Ewings in the UK to postulate the existence of aphasia in children and to try to find positive ways of identifying and treating it. The difficulty of making a positive identification is shown by cases of children who have had their diagnoses changed several times (Morley, 1973; Browning, 1987). A number of children has been shown to suffer from high frequency hearing loss in addition to developmental aphasia which made diagnosis doubly difficult.

Major attention has long been focused upon children who show abnormal responses to sound since these have become associated with continuing difficulties in comprehending or processing spoken language (Taylor, 1964; Worster-Drought, 1965). While the distinction between impaired auditory acuity and language disorder has become theoretically clear, it remains difficult to demonstrate in practice, particularly with extremely young children. Procedures for differential diagnosis are regularly revised and advocated (Ward and McCartney, 1978; Ward and Kellett, 1982; Ward, 1984).

The need to differentiate between those children who were generally retarded in all aspects of cognition and those who were language disordered was stimulated by advances in both fields. The opening up of the whole field of mental handicap in the last two decades has emphasized the importance of language in all aspects of teaching and training. This has led to better methods of assessment of language potential. Advances in linguistic knowledge and the awareness of how language is used in intelligence testing has shown us more clearly how language-disordered children may be penalised by such tests. Differentiation between the two groups is being made possible by the development of progressively refined and sophisticated measures of intelligence. However, considerable caution is necessary still in interpreting such measures because of the complex relationship between cognitive and linguistic ability. To some extent, children's responses to sensitive teaching are an excellent guide to their overall intellectual ability. But if their language disorders are not recognised, the wrong demands may be placed upon them and their potential left unrealised.

Differentiation between autism and language disorder, or more specifi-cally the aphasic type of language disorder, has received the continuous attention of Rutter and his colleagues (Rutter, Bartak and Newman, 1971;

Bartak, Rutter and Cox, 1975; Rutter, 1984; Rutter and Lord, 1987). Their investigations have illuminated both conditions. The distinction between the groups is a difficult one to make because of the frequency of overlapping symptoms. The type of language disorder most frequently confused with autism at the present time is that where the children show semantic–pragmatic difficulties. These are shown in the case history of the child Toni by Conti-Ramsden and Gunn (1986), and also the child Jonathan in Byers Brown and Beveridge (1979). The quest for differentiation between the two groups owes as much to scholarly as to remedial demands since the conditions are still imperfectly understood.

Presenting symptoms or abnormal behaviours which have prompted investigations into all these groups are recorded in a number of case studies written for both professional and non-professional readers (Greene, 1962; West, 1969; Wallace, 1986; Browning, 1987).

Normal and abnormal language acquisition

The slow emergence of linguistic features is a recognised characteristic of language disorder. Research and teaching efforts during the last decade have enabled us to document these features much more accurately then was previously possible. Conspicuous in this field is the work of Crystal who, together with colleagues, pioneered and propagated the linguistic profile (Crystal, Fletcher and Garman, 1976; Crystal, 1982b). This has many advantages over previous methods of representing the child's language level because it identifies the imbalances or mismatches between linguistic systems. It is consequently possible to distinguish at an early age between overall delay affecting all aspects of language and specific delays affecting one or more systems.

Menyuk in the USA was one of the first to draw attention to the importance of documenting the rate of linguistic feature acquisition and her early work on phonology has been followed by the major studies of Ingram in the USA (1974, 1976, 1987) and Grunwell in the UK (1975, 1980b, 1981). At the same time, interest was developing in measuring the other components of language namely grammatical structure, vocabulary acquisition and use, functional or interpersonal use of language. The last item was temporarily submerged in the 1960s and 1970s while more exact structural measurements were being pursued. It was brought into prominence in the UK through the work of Halliday (1975) and also through the studies of the American psychologist Bruner during his sojourn in Oxford (Bruner, 1983a,b). The attention this functional or pragmatic aspect of language has subsequently received has more than made amends for any temporary neglect. It has been greatly stimulated by research into infant behaviour and mother–child interaction. From such research findings it is possible to record both the normal interactions which prepare the way for intercourse through language and the abnormal interactions which delay this intercourse.

Writers in the 1970s were considerably occupied with the distinction between delayed and deviant development of spoken language. Byers Brown writing in 1976 expressed one view in the following way (it was previously pointed out that 'speech' is here synonymous with 'spoken language'):

> Delayed speech involves the late appearance of words and their combination into phrases and sentences. Rudimentary utterance and general behaviour may be on normal lines but the speech is less mature and less accomplished than is considered appropriate for the child's age or common among his peers. The utterance would be suitable to a younger child and could be found in the normal developmental sequence. The delay may also be apparent in the child's phonology or in his use of speech to control his environment.
>
> Deviant speech does not fit into a normal developmental sequence. It may manifest itself in voice or tone quality, sound structure or sound sequence. While gross deviations are likely to be associated with pathology, deviant phonological or syntactical constructions can occur in the absence of pathology, suggesting that the child is having difficulty in making deductions from the stream of sounds he hears or that he is not able to make use of his deductions to build up his language system in a conventional manner.

These conclusions were based upon the study of a clinical population considered retrospectively. They were not necessarily shared by investigators conducting research across large groups of language-delayed children. Some investigators considered that the term 'deviant' was never appropriate to developing language which contained phonemes and other linguistic structures which were normally produced but which occurred late or in unusual combination. [For further discussion of the use of 'delayed' and 'deviant' language, see Menyuk and Looney (1972) and Leonard (1972).]

At the present time Byers Brown's description of 'delayed speech' might be subsumed under 'immature' or 'transient' delays and her 'deviant speech' under true delay leading to disorder. We appear to circle around the position that there is a group of children whose speech appears late or emerges slowly but which improves spontaneously and another group sharing the same broad characteristics but which does not improve. We know a great deal more about the large heterogeneous group which does not improve but we remain in the frustrating position of being able to identify both groups only in retrospect, i.e. when improvement has or has not taken place. There is also the question of whether or not our follow-up studies take all the possible manifestations of language disorder into account or whether they still continue to think in terms of speech improvement. Another factor which is much better considered now is the possible extent of normal variation within language acquisition. We are now aware that although normal children master the same language skills they may adopt different strategies in order to do so. The more we know about these different strategies, the more we must question a simple division into normal and subnormal language acquisition.

It might seem as though we had made no progress in the first two of the three approaches toward differentiating language disorders from other behaviour or conditions. In fact, the position is much more encouraging and much more interesting today than previously. We have a much richer and more extensive database upon which to make our conclusions. The interdisciplinary nature of present investigations means that we are not only gaining in understanding of language disorders but of other forms of handicap concurrently.

Differentiation between different groups or subtypes

The first differentiation between subgroups of conditions in which language failed to emerge normally was between receptive and expressive conditions. Each of these was then examined for further distinctions. One of the first attempts at subtype differentiation by a British speech therapist was that of Greene (1963). Taking the broadly expressive group of disorders, Greene described one set of children whose delayed speech was associated with coordination disorder and another where there was language learning difficulty. Cooper and Griffiths (1978) subsequently presented a broad classification drawn from a sample of several hundred 6-year-old children with 'developmental dysphasia'. This was to be seen as a simple classification based upon the way the children presented in the classroom. All the children were free from major mental or physical handicaps. The classification contains five categories:

1. Children who demonstrate normal hearing upon audiometry but who show little or no ability to comprehend or use speech.
2. Children with varying degrees of hearing loss who have failed to respond to the use of sound amplification and the normal methods of teaching the deaf in that they have not acquired comprehension or use of spoken language.
3. Children with normal or near normal comprehension but with absence or severe retardation of spoken language.
4. A similar group to (3) but one in which spoken language shows a late onset (3–4 years) and then develops rapidly with only residual traces

of difficulty at 7–8 years. However, these children show severe reading difficulties.

5. Children who develop a grasp of the mechanics of speech but whose use is often imitative, stereotyped and irrelevant.

The authors describe each category fully in their text. They emphasise that there is overall diversity with gradations occurring within and between groups. The behaviour which they cover will doubtless appear in the subgroups made by a number of other authors. These will be presented in Chapter 7. The search for differential patterns of language as well as of behaviour has occupied a number of investigators. Notable among these are Aram and Nation who undertook a study of 47 children with developmental language disorders with the object of providing language performance data on an aetiologically heterogeneous sample. They arrived at a classification which they refer to as being clinically useful and meaningful to themselves but which would also have to emerge from other databases in the form of similar patterns. It is possible that the patterns which they identified and classified were the result of the specific battery of tests employed.

This observation by Aram and Nation highlights the difficulty in generalising from any one study, no matter how large or well controlled. Results may well reflect the skill and interest of the investigator rather than giving an accurate picture of the entire population. The refinement of categories within the population does not necessarily teach us more about the range and extent of the disorder although it appears to be an advance on individual clinical observation.

What happens to these children?

There are very good reasons to continue investigating language disorders on the lines indicated above. Among the most cogent is the hope that such investigations will result in better understanding and more effective management. If children's difficulties can be identified early and the course of the condition predicted, remedy can be channelled in the most efficient way. Studies to date have shown that there is a core of language-disordered children who go on to become learning disabled. Whether specialist intervention at one level can result in reduction of impairment at another remains speculative. The effects of therapy in altering the course of a language disorder have not been measured in large numbers because the course of language disorders is only now starting to be clarified. Investigators to date have been unable to affirm the positive effects of therapy in predicting outcome. Bishop and Edmundson (1987a,b) are among other authors in wishing to make it clear that strong conclusions about therapy effectiveness should not be drawn from their findings on this point. Their emphasis is proper and thoughtful since speech therapy in the UK has suffered from well-intentioned but premature attempts to evaluate its effectiveness. There is the need to be accountable and to be seen to be accountable which is recognised by the whole profession. The public must be assured that the help given to the handicapped, help which costs the public money, is the most effective that can be devised. Speech therapists are under the obligation to reduce the effects of any potentially handicapping condition to the greatest extent possible. They are not, however, under the obligation to cure conditions which arise from some essential flaw in the mechanism. Society does not require this of those who practise medicine nor should it require it of those who work in the remedial and caring professions. What society does require is skilled and expert treatment from professionals that will help individual sufferers to realise their potential, compensate for their handicaps and live happily with themselves. The community must play a full part then in the social adjustment of the handicapped population. It will be easier for society to do this when professionals are more fully committed to a proselytising role on behalf of their clientele. Since this must stem from knowledge and commitment rather than emotional appeal, we are brought back to the need for clear thinking, comprehensive description and accurate prediction.

There are not very many follow-up studies which offer real guidance to clinicians in where to place their emphasis. One of the most frequently quoted in the UK is that of Griffiths (1969) because her population, which was taken from a special school for language-disordered children, was clearly defined. Griffiths followed up these children after they had left the special school and had moved into various kinds of other educational provision. Among the more distressing of her findings was that, in spite of the carefully documented reports compiled for the guidance of teachers inheriting these children, the information had not been passed on to them. Twenty years later, identical findings are reported from speech therapists trying to follow-up individual children (Mobley, 1988, unpublished data).

Individual speech therapists who have practised for many years have tried to find out what has happened to the young language-disordered children with whom they worked. In the case of one of the authors of this text (BBB), the search has been conducted on both sides of the Atlantic. There is, of course, a great variation in the success and happiness the children have experienced. Among the observations reported by parents and friends, the following tend to reoccur. 'He doesn't have many friends, I would describe him as a loner.' 'He doesn't have a girl friend yet; I think girls find him rather immature.' Sometimes therapists are able to observe for themselves behaviour which brings home to them the full extent of 'residual disabilities' they may have been inclined to dismiss. A spouse may report that someone has telephoned but the message was difficult to understand. The caller turns out to be one of the best graduates from the language unit. Or, watching an adolescent girl dancing at a party may suddenly reveal the full extent of her motor coordination difficulties. Signs of fatigue remind one of how tiring it must be to spend the whole day concentrating hard to pick up information that most of us gather in passing. A mother speaks of the tantrums her 20-year-old son will still display if interrupted while watching television because he will not then be able to understand what is happening. These are the kinds of deficits shown by the language-disordered population which distinguishes it far more effectively from the low-verbal section of the normal population than do broad measures of verbal ability (Snyder, 1982).

Follow-up studies, whether individual or large and standardised, will continue to throw up questions as to the nature of provision for children with language disorders. Most countries seem to arrive at provision which includes individual therapy, unit or special class placement and special school placement. The nature of this provision will be examined more closely in Chapter 7. The major difficulty encountered in the UK is the need to share provision between health and education. Speech therapy services are organised under the National Health Service and there is no service category of 'teacher–therapist'. Nor indeed has there been any real attempt to train teachers to work with children who have language disorders. Only one course is at present offered to equip teachers for this role and it requires secondment which local education authorities are reluctant to provide. Some promise for the future is offered by a course which is now being planned as a joint venture between a school of speech therapy in a polytechnic and a neighbouring university department of education. The proposal is to develop a distance learning course to equip teachers to work with children suffering from severe speech and language problems (College of Speech Therapists, 1989).

In the USA, provision for all handicapped children and infants is made through the state education service. Teachers are trained to work with all groups of handicapped children including those who are communicatively impaired or learning disabled. However, in order to qualify for this provision, children must be registered as 'handicapped'. Many parents of preschool children object to such registration. Their only resource is to seek therapy through the private sector.

As our knowledge of language disorder increases, it is to be hoped that it will have a more pronounced and positive impact upon the flexible and continuous nature of service provision. In the meantime, it is important to prevent administrators from pinning provision to specific diagnoses or test results since these may be no better guides than the thoughtful results of experienced personnel. A final responsibility of professionals towards their clients is to make as sure as they can that professional services are employed to maximum advantage.

Chapter 2
Identification

Summary

This chapter surveys the ways in which language disorder can be identified. It considers some of the ideas which have been presented on both causal and associated factors with emphasis upon the part these play in identification. The multifactorial nature of language disorder is illustrated and the identification process is discussed. Early screening methods are examined and some evaluation made as to their merits and disadvantages. Particular attention is paid to the things that must be considered when trying to predict language disorders from early language delay. The findings from a multicentre US project on early identification are reported with some discussion as to the relative merits of screening instruments and parental report.

How can these children be found?

The prevailing philosophy of therapeutic intervention is that it should start as early as possible. There are many humane arguments to be used in support. The earlier a child is helped to come to terms with his disability, the more likely he is to find ways in which to help himself. The earlier the parents are given help and support, the more likely is the whole family to behave positively and hopefully. The earlier that education authorities are informed as to potential needs for special provision, the more chance there is of that provision being available. The sooner acquainted everyone in the child's environment is with his abilities and his needs, the easier it will be for him to receive encouragement and acceptance. The validity of these arguments, together with the economic factors upon which they impinge, will be discussed more thoroughly in Chapter 7. If they have any validity at all, however, then early identification, which logically precedes intervention, must take place as soon as possible.

There are also academic arguments to support the need for early identification. The sooner a condition is properly noted and described the better will be the chances of tracking its course. This will increase understanding. It has not been easy for past investigators to distinguish between the effects of the underlying condition itself and those effects which come about as the child tries to help or to protect himself from failure. The withdrawal, aggression and hyperactivity which some children show are only three of the behaviours which can make approach more difficult. There are many aspects of the children's behaviour which can compound their difficulties either through disguising the basic deficiency or by antagonising those who try to help them. If we are to understand how language disorders develop, we need to know how they start.

It has been pointed out (Byers Brown, 1987) that our ideas as to what constitutes early identification are under constant revision as our knowledge accrues. Two decades ago we would have been thinking about the 3 year old. Now, our interest in emergent language and our greatly increased knowledge in all aspects of child development make us look for signs of abnormality during the period when normal language is acquired, i.e. the first 3 years of life. We also know more about the factors that place a child at risk for developmental disorders in the biological sense and of those environmental and social circumstances which compound the risk. We may therefore start to identify developmental language disorders by looking at the settings in which they are most likely to be found.

It would be misleading to suggest that language disorders are only identified in infancy or early childhood. The identification may be made by the class teacher who realises that the difficulty a pupil is having in learning to read is outside the range of normal variation. Identification may come about through a social worker who perceives antisocial behaviour in an adolescent as stemming from basic communication problems. We cannot hope to identify all developmental language disorders at the time when the bases of language are being laid down even though this must be our aim. So all parents and professionals must be encouraged to understand how the disorders may manifest themselves. This aspect of public education will be considered more thoroughly in the next chapter.

What do we know about these children?

Family history

There is a large repository of clinical record to support the familial factor in developmental language disorder. Students have been trained to obtain a family history of language abilities and disabilities since systematic clinical training began. Individual therapists offer evidence of families which have yielded several members to their care. Some of the longer serving have worked with two generations of language-disordered children. Investigators have long observed an apparent familial component to developmental language disorders. What have been lacking are methodologies for investigation and clear indications as to aetiology. There is reason to suppose that these lacks may be remedied.

The first textbook devoted to genetic aspects of speech and language disorders was published in 1983 (Ludlow and Cooper, 1983). Figures on familial incidence are starting to become available. Edwards quotes from the findings of a multicentre study (Edwards *et al.*, 1984) involving 187 children with ages from 3 to 6 years. These children were referred from the regular clinic clientele of participating therapists with a diagnosis of 'language disorder' and no other significant handicaps. Of the 187 children, 55% of the boys and 39% of the girls had blood relatives with some kind of speech disability. This figure prompted the author to speculate that, if a genetic factor is involved, boys are more vulnerable.

Both Robinson (1987) and Sonksen (1979) found risk factors in familial conditions to be higher in boys than in girls. The highest risk is for brothers of boys and the lowest for sisters of girls. Robinson studied the records of children from Moor House School, a residential school for children with severe disorders of speech and language. From this population, he quotes a total figure of 40% for children with some positive family history, 28% having a parent or sibling affected. Robinson (1987), in a useful table, shows accordance between these figures and those of Sonksen. There is fair accordance with the earlier findings of Ingram (1959, 1965) and with Edwards more recent figures for less severely affected children. The presumption is that there is a genetic factor operating in both severe and moderate language disorders but as yet aetiology with a single locus has not been revealed. The fact that even though siblings may show language disorders they are not necessarily as severe as those shown by the target child, is only one indication of the complex nature of the aetiology.

All investigators in language disorder report a higher incidence in males than females. The Isle of Wight study (Rutter, Tizard and Whitmore, 1970) found a ratio of 6.2% : 4% in a population of 5 year olds. Sheridan (1973), reporting on the findings from the 7-year cohort of the National Children's Bureau Study, gives a ratio of 2 : 1 in favour of the males. Edwards reports a figure of 3 : 1 in the same direction and explains this higher ratio by referring to the younger age of her sample. She quotes Morley's (1957) original finding from the 1000 family study in Newcastle which showed that male children developed speech more slowly than did female children. This leads Edwards to surmise that maturational delay in part accounted for the disproportion between her findings and those of other investigators.

A number of possible contributory factors to the higher incidence of more severe and persistent disorders in males is discussed by Satz and Zaide in the Ludlow and Cooper text (1983).

The evidence on familial incidence of developmental disorder may help identification in a broad epidemiological sense but cannot necessarily be expected to pick up the individual child. We cannot assume that all parents will react with prompt concern to early signs of disordered language because they have experienced difficulties themselves or in other offspring. While it is likely that memories of their own distress will prompt them to seek help for their child earlier rather than later, it is also possible that the condition will cause less than usual concern because it is familiar. Parents' attitudes and beliefs will affect their behaviour quite as much as will their knowledge.

Research into family histories will help to identify the individuals who are most at risk but it is not likely to prevent the births of more at-risk infants. Although the penalties for language disorder can be very high, they are not the kind of penalties that prevent people from having children. If society becomes more helpful toward the communicatively impaired, there is likely to be more social and sexual intercourse among them. Consequently, the incidence of familial disorders may increase.

Chromosomal abnormalities

The preceding paragraph does not necessarily apply in those cases where language impairment is part of a syndrome giving rise to other major handicaps (e.g. Duchenne-type muscular dystrophy). Such conditions do not account for any substantial proportion of language disorders and neither do the chromosomal abnormalities which have been found in association with grossly delayed expressive speech. Garvey and Mutton selected 9 children from a pool of 450 with severe speech and language problems. These 9 children had normal comprehension for speech but grossly delayed expression. The children thus constituted a special subtype. Of the nine cases studied, three showed chromosomal abnormalities (Garvey and Mutton, 1973). Robinson gives a figure of 3–5% of all children with developmental language disorders as having some kind of chromosomal abnormalities. This figure is based upon several different studies. Follow-up studies of infants found on newborn screening to have chromosomal abnormalities, reveal that about half of these infants show delay in language development or show speech problems. Robinson, again basing his deductions on the results of a number of studies, says that the communication problems are most consistantly demonstrated in boys with Klinefelter's syndrome but are also seen in XYY boys. However, not all children with these chromosomal abnormalities show delayed language development nor is it always severe and persistent in those who do so. The fragile-X chromosome syndrome has been associated with delayed language development although the relationship between the two has yet to be thoroughly explored. It appears likely that the delay in language may be part of a general developmental delay rather than one focused upon language.

A medically based aetiology

The search for one main causative factor which can be revealed through medical examination has not been productive. The consensus of opinion is that there is no one overriding aetiology. Nevertheless there are factors which medical examination cannot overlook since they have been shown to be associated with delayed or abnormal language development. Careful examination must be made to exclude the two main causes of language delay in children, namely hearing loss and general intellectual impairment. The most likely common factor between language disorders which is not associated with these two groups is some degree of neurological impairment. Language disorders have been shown to coexist with mild types of cerebral palsy and with clumsiness. It is reasonable to look toward a damaged nervous system to unite the many different perceptual–motor problems which are encountered in the language-disordered population. The possible roles of brain abnormalities and brain damage are discussed by Goodman in a recent text (1987). He observes that: 'At present, the hypothesis that all developmental language disorders have a neurological basis is attractive but unproven.'

Goodman states that neurological explanations tend to fall into one of three groups: maturational lag, atypical lateralisation and focal abnormality.

Maturational lag

The theory of maturational lag is appealing to many since, as Goodman points out: 'Everyday experience teaches us that children mature at different rates and that the same child may mature quickly in one area and slowly in another'. Rutter (1984), in propounding the theory, suggests that 'unusually great variations in rates of brain maturation might be responsible for specific delays in the development of particular brain functions (such as speech or language)' (p. 584). The support for maturational lag as a general aetiology for language disorders is weak but authors indicate that it could account for some of them. The theory would be expected to account for those children who show early delays in language development but who eventually catch up with their peers. Stark, Mellits and Tallal (1983) discuss this group of language-delayed children and contrast them with a group considered to be severely language impaired. The language-impaired children are likely to present a number of deficits in perceptual and motor skills or a few very severe deficits. These deficits, together with the language impairment and possible difficulty in interacting with other people, could be associated with significant neurological impairment. The authors do not state the possible neurological association with language delay. They suggest that some of the skills underpinning language may not emerge sufficiently to contribute to the child's language learning at the usual time. Consequently there may be temporary but marked delay in that aspect of language. As the child perceives the nature and use of language more clearly, and as other aspects of the whole process appear, there may be acceleration of language development.

Bishop and Edmundson (1987a) have considered the distinction between the two groups made by Stark, Mellits and Tallal (1983) in light of their own research findings. This consideration prompted them to test out the hypothesis of maturational lag as it might apply to a language-delayed and a language-impaired group. They suggested that if the language-delayed children developed at a normal rate after a slow start, maintaining the same intervals between language milestones, the children 'would be aptly described as having maturational lag' (Bishop and Edmundson, 1987b). The language-impaired children should be characterised by slow rates of development with verbal skills plateauing early. Thus the theoretical position could be tested by testing the prediction that the rate of language development would be different between the groups. A second approach was to look for evidence of immaturity in the motor functioning of the language-delayed group. The authors cite Wolff, Gunnoe and Cohen (1985) that neuromotor measures provide reliable criteria for developmental age in young children. If the language-delayed children showed initial immaturity of neuromotor function with gradual improvement, it would be evidence of overall maturation. The language-impaired children would not be expected to show this improvement since they were considered to have more significant neuropathology. Bishop and Edmundson failed to find differentiating factors between the two groups on the lines anticipated. There was no distinctive difference in the rate of progress made by the children when assessed at intervals by a verbal test battery. Nor was it possible to differentiate between the groups on the grounds of simple motor maturation. The investigators concluded that both subgroups seemed to be best accounted for in terms of brain maturation because both groups made steady progress after a delayed start. They note problems which challenge the maturational lag hypothesis as a general aetiology, however. These concern the uneven pattern of language impairment which is not indicative of immaturity; also the logical fact that if maturational lag rather than neurological impairment is present, children should eventually catch up rather than show persisting problems in a number of language and language-related skills.

Atypical lateralisation

The literature on cerebral lateralisation in relation to disorders of language and fluency is considerable and controversial. Even granted the coexist-ence of some of the phenomena, it is not possible to tease out cause and effect. For example, does developmental language disorder arise from atypical patterns of cerebral lateralisation or do both conditions arise from an underlying brain abnormality? Robinson essays a unifying hypothesis based upon cerebral lateralisation which he considers accounts for a number of apparently disparate observations about specific developmental language disorders. The hypothesis is based upon the work of Geschwind and Galaburda. Robinson suggests that most observations on causal factors in developmental language disorder can be accounted for in terms of asymmetry of brain structure and function, with the left hemisphere destined to be responsible for: language and certain fine motor skills in most individuals; genetic and intrauterine environmental influences upon this left hemisphere specialisation; the slow maturation of the left hemisphere in relation to the right, notably in males; the increased vulnerability of the brain to adverse influences during maturation which is again more marked in males; genetic and environmental influences which act upon the maturing brain. The interaction of the above factors can account for the higher proportion of males than females among the developmentally disordered. It can also account for the proportion of other neurological abnormalities which is higher in the language-disordered than in the normal population.

There is no real quarrel between this kind of thinking and the concept of maturational lag. One could suggest that the difference between the delayed and impaired group of children, both suggested by Bishop and Edmundson to show this lag, is in the extent of the adverse impacts upon the maturing brain. Identification of language disorder (comprehending both delay and impairment) must continue to take firm account of the timing and rate of early language emergence.

Focal abnormalities

Focal abnormalities have been cited as a possible cause for the failure of development of particular skills. There is not an extensive literature upon this subject although it will doubtless continue to grow as examinations become more refined. Presumably the plasticity of the infant brain and its capacity to recover from insult would also be a factor in compensation for focal abnormality. Of extreme importance to language development would be the time when any such lesion occurs. (For discussion of recovery from brain damage see Goodman (1987) and for review of the evidence for acquired lesions early in life as a cause of language disorder see Bishop (1987a).)

Even if neurological factors are not responsible for all cases of disordered language in developing children, they appear sufficiently frequently to make all infants at risk for abnormal neurological development also at risk for abnormal language development.

Perinatal factors

One population of infants that is held to be at risk for neurological impairment is the premature or pre-term population and particularly babies of very low birth weight. These babies should therefore be followed up at regular intervals to see that their language, among other skills, is developing normally. Evidence to date has been contradictory. Stevenson, Bax and Stevenson (1982) found no statistically significant association between either the gestational age of the child or the birth weight and speech and language delay at the age of three, although there was a non-significant trend in the expected direction. Bax (1987) considers that the relationship is still unclear and reminds us that since both low birth weight and speech and language delay are common in most developed countries, chance associations will occur.

Wright *et al.* (1983) found a significant difference between the language status of low birth weight and normal infants when assessed at 3;5 years. Byers Brown, Bendersky and Chapman (1986) also found a significant delay in the development of the speech–sound system in pre-term infants as compared with the normal population. The trend was more marked in infants who had sustained intraventricular haemorrhage (IVH), the range of delay being wider. On the other hand, Menyuk, Liebergott and Schultz (1986) found no significant differences in the lexical or phonological development of premature and full-term infants when measures were taken at intervals during the second and third years of life.

The above findings turn out to be less contradictory when all of the associated variables have been examined. Wright *et al.* emphasize the importance of social and environmental factors in influencing language development and thus helping infants to achieve normal language levels in their preschool years despite the initial effects of prematurity. Byers Brown, Bendersky and Chapman (1986) express considerable caution about the predictive value of their findings. In fact, subsequent research (Lewis and Bendersky, 1989) has shown that the number of medical complications correlated most highly with language skill whether or not IVH had occurred. The authors suggest that development of the pre-term child be studied with an interactional view of various factors such as medical complications and socioeconomic status which could have an impact upon each other. This point had been raised in a paper by D'Souza *et al.* (1981) in a study of 26 survivors of perinatal asphyxia when examined between the ages of 2 and 5 years. Nine of these children showed speech and language deficits independent of physical or mental handicap. D'Souza *et al.* indicate that the relationship between environmental factors and speech and language development had not been adequately established with regard to perinatal conditions and that in some cases the origin of the language delay was multifactorial.

Menyuk, in discussing her results, suggested that the children who were showing normal language levels at the preschool stage might show difficulty later when language became more complex (a possibility that must presumably be extended to children in the other studies cited). Moreover, Menyuk's subjects were not drawn from lower socioeconomic groups. What emerges from these studies of at-risk infants is that factors can be noted at different age points which may or may not signal deviations from normal patterns. However, in order to assess the importance of any one factor, such as prematurity, the possible influence of many circumstances which are associated with it (single parent status, poverty, malnutrition) have to be teased out and separately considered as by Lewis and Bendersky. Since very low birth weight children are now the recipients of regular follow-up programmes in a number of countries, not only should early identification of language disorders be facilitated but the course of the disorders should be illuminated.

It will be apparent from the discussion so far that while certain medical and environmental factors may place children at risk for language disorder, they do not, in themselves, identify. Language disorders can only be identified as language emerges or fails to emerge. Moreover, at the emergent stage there is no guarantee that the signs will be stable. Byers Brown (1987) quotes from a follow-up investigation of one of the IVH children in the 1986 study. When first assessed, the child was 16 months of age or 13 months corrected age. Findings were as follows:

Bayley Scales of Mental and Motor Development	Mental scale	69
	Motor scale	99
Sequenced Inventory of Communication Development	Receptive age	8 months
	Expressive age	12 months
Speech–sound estimate		9 months

The picture appeared to be one of cognitive and linguistic delay with strengths on the motor side. However, when reassessed at the age of 3;4 years, the balance had shifted.

Stanford Binet Intelligence Scales	Test composite	95
Sequenced Inventory of Communicative Ability	Receptive age	36 months
	Expressive age	36 months

The mean length of utterance (MLU) calculated from a spontaneous speech sample gave an age equivalent of 35 months. This child would no longer be considered as language or cognitively delayed. Although on the low side of average, he is not significantly retarded. At the same time he is recorded as showing some movement disorder and his speech is not easily intelligible due to immature articulation. At this age he appears to be showing more difficulty with motor than with other skills. His case illustrates the caution which must be shown in predicting the course of language development in very young, damaged infants. The capacity of the nervous system to recover from insult sustained at an early age must be taken into account. It will be necessary to assess this child in the future to make sure that he has escaped language disorder but his position at 3 years is heartening.

Other causal correlates

Otitis media

Otitis media became a prime contender for the role of chief causal agent in developmental language disorders as we moved into the 1980s. It had been demonstrated as early as 1970 (Owrid, 1970; Hamilton and Owrid, 1974) that the conductive hearing loss resulting from otitis media depressed verbal skills and educational attainments in school children. During the following decade attention became focused upon the effects of recurrent episodes of otitis media on the child's developing linguistic system. Anxiety was not only generated by evidence of sustained conductive loss but by the number of early episodes of otitis media suffered by the child. The broad questions posed were:

● Does otitis media lead to language disorder?
● Does otitis media always lead to conductive loss and thence to language delay?

Since otitis media is episodic and associated with fluctuations in hearing, children who encountered a number of episodes during their early development were deemed to be at particular risk in the acquisition of phonology and syntax. Fluctuating hearing losses in the region of 40 dB would mean that the infant failed to hear a number of important auditory/linguistic clues (e.g. tense, plurality). By causing confusion because of its fluctuations, the condition would prevent the acquisition of good listening skills which might allow the child to compensate. However, the otitis media argument was not just based upon the possible relationship between fluctuations in hearing and delays in mastering language structure.

In the USA, deductions were made from the results of animal experiments and these were then transferred to the human infant. Experimental studies using animals showed that deprivation of auditory stimulation could lead to atrophy of auditory function. It was then hypothesised that the effect of otitis media in infancy might be such as to cause recurrent conductive loss with consequent failure of the function of hearing to develop. This failure of development could not be compensated for by subsequent restoration to health of the middle ear. This theory was effectively challenged by Ventry (1980) and was subsequently replaced by studies which were more immediately related to the practical effects of conductive loss during the period of language learning. There have been a number of reviews of the role of otitis media as a long-term influence upon language development (Paradise, 1981; Bishop, 1986; Hasenstab, 1987) and a very large number of studies exploring the relationship (Jerger *et al.*, 1983; Shriberg and Smith, 1983; Teele *et al.*, 1984). Attention has been directed to both comprehension and production of the language system and on both disorders and delays. Since the comprehension of spoken language depends upon the ability to hear a number of unstressed syllables and low energy, low volume sounds, it is logical to deduce that a fluctuating hearing loss which reduced this ability could be responsible for both delay and disorder. Since the ability to generate a sound system depends on knowledge of the sounds which are required by that system, it is also logical to attribute system failure to faulty information based upon hearing impairment.

Practising clinicians are as likely to be swayed in their judgements of the effects of otitis media by the children they treat as they are by research studies. Most speech therapists working with young children can cite instances where periods of conductive loss interfered markedly with a child's language learning. As speech therapists do not see children with otitis media, conductive loss and normal speech, they are not in a position to make judicial statements as to the importance of otitis media as a causal factor. Byers Brown (1981) cites the cases of three male children seen in the clinic during their fourth year of age. Each boy showed evidence of conductive hearing loss. In the first case, the diagnosis was of delayed speech and language and this was resolved within months of medical treatment which restored hearing to the normal level. In the second case the diagnosis of delayed language was complicated by hyperactivity and attentional problems leaving the role of conductive loss unclear. In fact, restoration of normal middle ear function was not followed by language improvement but by echolalia, continuing attentional difficulties and general linguistic immaturity. This would appear to be a case where the language disorder was primary and the hearing loss compounding.

The third child showing conductive hearing loss was also diagnosed as having a general developmental delay. However, good cognitive ability was revealed both through assessment and through observation and parental report. Speech was severely retarded. Treatment to alleviate the conductive hearing loss again restored normal middle ear function. There was no immediate increase in spoken language but progress in that area was steady

Table 2.1 Otitis media and developmental language disorder

Child	Age (years)	Presenting symptom	Hearing	Speech–language	Treatment	Outcome
Child A	3;8	Delayed speech	a/c loss 40–45 dB R 45 dB L b/c 5–10 dB Speech discrimination: Kendall Toy Test 50/55 dB Impedance showed poor compliance with negative middle ear pressures of −250 mmHg	Immature phonology and syntax Hyponasal voice quality	Adenoidectomy Myringotomy Language stimulation with focus on listening; auditory discrimination; vocabulary sentence expansion	Normal hearing Age appropriate syntax Resolving phonological immaturities Normal voice quality
Child B	3;3	Delayed speech Temper tantrums, hyperactivity	Variable responses to sounds but mainly 55–60 dB Would not allow impedance testing; subsequent otological examination revealed fluid	Immaturity in all aspects of language plus attention difficulty	Adenoidectomy and myringotomy Language stimulation plus attention control	Auditory behaviour still variable; broad scatter of responses to language assessment suggestive of primary language disorder
Child C	3;9	Delayed speech and delayed motor development	a/c 50 dB R and L b/c normal Impedance curves very flat with poor compliance and negative pressure	Severe retardation of expressive language with good comprehension	Tonsilectomy; adenoidectomy and myringotomy Language therapy with focus upon imitation, sound production discrimination, modelling and sentence expansion	Normal hearing Continued language therapy with emphasis on syntax until 5;0 years when performance was age appropriate

and sustained. Verbal comprehension was within normal for age limits by the end of 6 months and verbal expression within a year. In this case, the hearing loss was also considered to be a compounding rather than a causal factor. The delayed language development was probably consequent upon maturational lag affecting a number of skills.

The case histories of the three boys are summarised in Table 2.1. Individual case histories of this kind cannot be expected to resolve the broad questions posed at the start of this section. What they can do is to remind us of the need to explore the child's hearing levels and auditory behaviour before and during any treatment for delayed language. The significance of a conductive loss in relation to language development will vary according to the child's other abilities and deficits. Most investigators are convinced of the multifactorial nature of language disorders. While results of many of the investigations of otitis media and language disorder are inconclusive, few would be prepared to discount the possible adverse effects when combined with other predisposing factors. The weight of statistical evidence emerging from any forthcoming study of the relationship between otitis media, conductive hearing loss and language disorder should not interfere with the scrupulous appraisal of this relationship in any one child.

Cognitive impairment

The relationship between cognitive and language development is of major interest in attempting to specify the presence and the nature of a language disorder. The emergence of a child's first words has always been held to reveal his ability to think. First words are therefore a source of gratification and relief to parents and of particular interest to psychologists. Children who show delay in the onset of words and particularly word combinations may also show difficulties in verbal comprehension. Such children are likely to be at risk for general cognitive impairment particularly if they also show delay in the acquisition of motor skills. The more a child's delay is focused upon one aspect of linguistic development, the more likely he is to be heading for a language, rather than a general intellectual, problem. However, this is to make only the broadest and simplest statement about the relationship. Language disorders may be so pervasive that they affect the developing child's ability to acquire verbal symbols and insightful language strategies. As a consequence his ability to demonstrate normal thought processes will be affected.

There is a very considerable body of work devoted to the development of both cognition and language and to their relative dependence or independence. The influence of this literature has been felt in both the diagnosis and remediation of language handicap. Early diagnoses tended to rest upon the discrepancy between verbal and non-verbal skills as demonstrated by intelligence tests. As the child grew older, tests became more heavily loaded verbally. So children who had been thought to be 'within normal limits' intellectually were found to show relatively low overall functioning in relation to their peers. Many questions arose from such results. The tests themselves were subjected to stringent criticism, the nature of language in problem solving was examined, and the performance of language-disordered children on a large number of cognitive processing tasks was explored.

Rice (1983), in a helpful review, indicates the bewildering array of studies through which language-disordered children were found to perform more poorly than their peers with normal language and refers to a detectable sense of frustration regarding the elusiveness of cognition and its role in language impairment and of the remediation process. This kind of frustration was suffered by those in research more than by those in therapy where the interest and stimulation from cognitive exploration was very positive in its effects. The main focus was upon the very young child. Language therapists grasped the idea of early symbolic function as a vital precursor to language function. If symbolic activity was present in one domain, e.g. play, it not only indicated the potential for cognitive development but the possibility of transfer to another domain, that of verbal symbols. Play became a highly important diagnostic and therapeutic tool in the preschool language clinic. While the benefits were considerable in many associated areas, mother—child interaction, concentration and general well being, there was little research from the clinical side to affirm the transfer from one form of symbolic activity to another. Largo and Howard (1979) point out that the relationship between play behaviour and language acquisition has turned out to be more complex than at first supposed. More recently, Thai and Bates (1988) have offered evidence in support of a local homology whereby specific impairments in play may predict specific patterns of early language impairment. The authors negate the idea of a common symbolic function underlying both skills. The diagnostic importance of play is likely to be increased rather than diminished by this suggestion.

Rice's paper explores the territory of linguistic and non-linguistic knowledge in relation to cognition. She shows that while each has its own domain, there is a sizeable area of overlap in which linkage is possible. The question of major interest is whether the language disordered experience most difficulty in the shared domain or in the territory peculiar to language. Benton (1978) in an earlier review looks at some of the evidence to support the view that dysphasia is the particular expression of a cognitive impairment affecting non-verbal as well as verbal behaviour. One such hypothesis deals with the processing of auditory information. This is a 'modal-specific' cognitive deficit and is indeed dealt with in the same volume (Tallal and Piercy, 1978) as a defect of auditory perception. We see here some of the difficulties confronting those who tried to separate auditory processing from other cognitive activities. Tests to demonstrate auditory processing difficulty could only be carried out by children who had achieved a fairly high level of cognitive function. Such testing therefore becomes specific cognitive testing and the hypothesis of an auditory sequencing impairment constituting the common denominator in language disorder cannot be upheld or refuted (for further discussion see Rees, 1973).

Generally speaking, the education of speech—language therapists has not equipped them for the cognitive exploration of language disorders which is now required. Little is known about the development of children's thinking. The present interest in pragmatic skills stimulates the need to find out how children become aware of other people in all sorts of contexts. Such awareness is known to be lacking in the language disordered. We have to ascertain the extent to which this lack of insight is the product of unrealistic teaching and therapy and how much is part of the language disability. There are many other aspects to be examined. For example Lloyd (1982) pointed out that when children are fully stretched by cognitive demands they have little energy left for monitoring the procedure. It may be that some of our procedures are too demanding for the children and their monitoring skills cannot develop as a consequence. These points will be considered more fully in the discussion on therapeutic intervention (see Chapter 7). So far as identification is concerned we may summarise the cognitive aspect as follows:

● Children who show delay in the acquisition of all aspects of language may be at risk for cognitive impairment.
● Children who show evidence of cognitive impairment will be at risk for language delay and may be at risk for language disorders.
● Delay in the emergence of symbolic play may herald either or both of the above conditions.
● Language disorder may be heralded by a drop in the achievements of children previously showing average attainments on intelligence testing.
● Language disorder may be indicated if children show considerable variability and quick fatigue in cognitive tasks.
● Language disorder is more likely to be associated with inconsistency and variability in learning than is overall cognitive impairment and is also more likely to be modality specific.

Several of these points are in accordance with Shatz's (1977) observation that children with limited capacity processing may show only sporadic grasp of certain skills.

Environmental risk factors

The identification of language disorders must involve examination of the factors in the child's environment which impede his learning of his native language. Attention must be paid to class and cultural considerations and the way in which these interact with biological risk factors. It has been many times stated that the factors that place children at risk for language disorder are compounds and not single entities. Children are placed at biological risk if they are born prematurely, if they are small for dates and if they are born to mothers who have taken drugs, smoked or drunk to excess during pregnancy. Poorly nourished, tired and worried mothers are far less likely to produce healthy infants than are those who are well cared for and well endowed. The materially developed countries of the Western World have reason to be very concerned about the numbers of infants being born into financially deprived environments and also into environments which are polluted and unhealthy.

Children born at biological risk may be further affected in their development by parental attitudes. Poorly educated parents are less able to take advantage of what is offered in the way of health care than those who are well read and well informed. Mothers who are chronically tired and harassed will not have the time and energy to enjoy their babies and to interact with them in the positive way that will prepare them for communication through language. Many infants at biological risk are the products of teenage pregnancies. Very young mothers may have emotional needs of their own which are too strong to allow them to see their infants as individual beings with needs peculiar to themselves. Environmental risks to child development can best be viewed within a cumulative framework. We should start from first principles, that infants thrive best when they are healthy, well cared for, wanted and enjoyed.

Sensory deprivation

Severe sensory deprivation which occurs when children are reared in severely abnormal circumstances will surely prevent the acquisition of language. The case most frequently cited in the literature of language pathology is that of Genie (Curtiss, 1977). Such tragic children cannot yield clear-cut evidence as to the effects of language deprivation alone since their chronic malnutrition prevents normal brain development.

Attempts to study the effects on children of lack of early stimulation have therefore focused upon those whose bodies have been reasonably well cared for but whose minds have been chronically understimulated. J.R. Edwards (1979) reviews some of the evidence for and against sensory deprivation as a component of social disadvantage in his text *Language and Disadvantage*. He goes on to review some of the wealth of literature generated in the 1950s and 1960s upon social deprivation and its relationship to educational retardation. At this time both the USA and the UK were concerned that children from low socioeconomic level, disadvantaged families might be permanently penalised. The well-known Head Start programme arose in the USA in the attempt to prepare such children for school by giving them a richer social experience at preschool level. Edwards (1979) points out that this programme and others were linguistically unsophisticated and it was only under the influence of sociolinguistic research and pressure that language was seen as the most important component of early social disadvantage.

Language disadvantaged and language different

The specific nature of 'Black Speech' received considerable attention in the USA first in relation to disadvantage and subsequently in relation to language difference. The distinction between the two is made by many authors and in particular Taylor (1982) has expanded upon it specifically in relation to speech–language pathology. Whereas it was originally posited that children raised within a Black culture might suffer from deficiencies of language form, it is now considered that 'Black Speech' is not grammatically incorrect but is subject to its own linguistic rules. Obviously children who are brought up within one language idiom and then educated within another could have initial difficulties. However, these do not need to be permanently penalising. Care is now being taken to ensure that Black children receive attention not only from teachers from their own culture but also from therapists and other professional workers. This being so, they are less likely to have behaviour which is normal to their culture construed as abnormal in terms of their development.

Black culture stands in a slightly different position to that of other minority groups since it is indigenous to the southern USA. Other minority groups in the USA and the UK are now bringing their own immigrant cultures. It is of first importance that children are assessed for possible language disorder in their own native language (*see* Chapter 6). Materials still need to be developed for this purpose and also for the assessment of children whose first language is Welsh. The concept of a multiracial, multicultural society may be accepted by professionals but the practicalities are slow to be worked out.

Social class

The multicultural society is more topical in professional discussion among speech therapists than is social class. The latter was the focus of much interest during the 1960s when Bernstein's ideas were widely commented upon and widely misconstrued. It was then considered likely that children who were brought up in working class environments were at a disadvantage compared to those middle class children who had been exposed to a richer and more formal language experience during their formative years. This was partly because the child was likely to be educated by middle class professionals no matter what his background. Children coming from middle class backgrounds were therefore deemed to have considerable early advantages. The permanent effect of early language disadvantage or difference (see Edwards, 1979) is now disproved in general terms. However, children who lack language stimulation in the sense of encouragement and enrichment are more likely to be delayed in language acquisition than are their linguistically privileged peers. This becomes a matter of some importance when instruments for language screening are being propagated.

Language opportunity and mother–child interaction

It is very generally reported that children who lack opportunity to talk with adults or who have to compete continually for adult attention may show language delay. Evidence is yielded by both twin studies (Savic, 1980) and by the literature on social deprivation (Edwards, 1979). One important variable in conducting research into language delay is the number of children in the home who are under 18 years of age. The British multicentre survey (M. Edwards, 1984) found that children with one or more siblings were over-represented in its sample when compared with the normal population distribution. Youngest children formed the majority of referrals. This finding was constant across all age groups within the sample range (3–6). The study did not find a higher incidence of referrals from one-parent families nor from families where the mother was employed outside the home. It is not possible to draw firm conclusions from these findings in the absence of information about child-minding arrangements.

Another aspect of interest is that of mother–child matching in the development of language strategies. Bruner (1983a,b) describes some early work on infant language learning. The mother is noted as capitalising upon an object or activity which attracts the infant's attention. She establishes a joint referrant for herself and her infant and makes this the focus of language, naming and describing. The development of this behaviour provides the language scaffolding through which the child can master linguistic forms by which to communicate experience. Bruner posits that the existence of a complex supportive language network, or Language Support System, makes possible the operation of genetically determined language devices.

A considerable literature has developed about the mother's behaviour in facilitating the language development of her child. A number of studies (Snow, 1972; Bloom, 1973; Snow and Ferguson, 1977) has shown how mothers adjust their speech to the developing abilities of their language-learning infants. Mothers produce speech which is syntactically simple, redundant and semantically related to topics of interest to young children. This simplified register has come to be known as 'motherese'. Authors have challenged the idea that children do in fact learn best from simplified data (Gleitman, Newport and Gleitman, 1984) and it has been suggested that language is most helpfully learned from data which mirror the range and complexities of the language system. Others (Furrow and Nelson, 1986) affirm the opposite view. The argument is obviously of more than academic interest to speech therapists both as regards the causal and the remedial aspects of speech delay. It has been demonstrated (Lieven, 1978) that there are conspicuous differences in the response parents make to conversationally adept and conversationally inept children. Handicapped children who cannot signal their intentions nor generate statements cannot stimulate adults to respond. Thus communication breaks down and with it the possibility of language growth. However, this is a long way from saying that normal children may become language deficient because their mothers fail to talk to them in an appropriate way.

At the present time (Summer 1988) there is research being generated on both sides of the Atlantic upon individual variation in child language learning and in maternal language. Many suppositions about factors making for language delay have been made without knowledge of individual variation. The question of language style and of style matching has yet to find a place in the literature of language therapy. Clinicians do not, as a matter of routine, analyse the language of adults when interacting with the infants and children in their care. We may hope to see more emphasis upon the dyad in future investigation. Conti-Ramsden (1987) has drawn attention to the importance of placing any dyadic analyses within the context in which they occur if a true picture is to emerge. Such analyses could then lead to interactive language therapy making use of each partner's contribution.

We will now turn from those factors which are important in identification to the manner in which the identification takes place.

Screening

Procedures for language screening must satisfy the ethical requirements laid down by the WHO (1980) and respected by all in health care. One absolute prerequisite is that the condition under identification is one that can be cured or mitigated and the second is that procedures exist for cure or remediation. When children are screened for language disorders we must ensure that special education and therapy are available. The step between screening and remediation is diagnosis to determine whether a condition which is handicapping does indeed exist. Assessment is the fellow of diagnosis since this shows the extent of the handicapping features together with the strengths and abilities which accompany them.

To screen is to administer a simple procedure that will accurately pick out children who may need special services. A screen will separate out those children who need further investigation from those whose development and attainments are normal or who are not at risk for the condition under investigation. Screening procedures must be:

- Economical both in time and materials.
- Simple and capable of being replicated by other professional workers.
- Comprehensive in the area of interest.
- Sufficiently accurate to ensure a minimum of false positives and false negatives, that is to say that they should be capable of detecting children who have the condition and not identifying those who do not.
- Cost effective – the condition to be detected must affect a large number of children whose progress as a result of early detection will save special medical and educational expenses such as to balance the costs of screening.

Any kind of identification procedure creates anxiety. People exposing themselves to medical screening of any kind must understand the consequences of identification. Women who submit themselves for breast or cervical cancer screening have been shown to react with considerable distress to findings that indicate they are at risk. It is highly important therefore that they should have immediate access to investigative and counselling services. However, they also have a responsibility to prepare themselves for screening by finding out as much as they can beforehand and making sure that they are able to tolerate an adverse result. Those involved in testing for AIDS may refuse to undertake the testing unless the subject has access to counselling. This is a major deterrent to demanding widespread screening for the condition in the general population. If the condition to be identified already involves a specialised population with access to guidance, quick screening may be carried out during routine follow-up procedures. If the question is whether or not to screen a large, normal and unsuspecting population, investigators must think very carefully about ethics and consequences.

All this may seem rather laboured in relation to a non-life-threatening condition such as language learning. Nevertheless, the argument is the same. If the condition is serious enough to demand early identification and investigation, it is sufficient to cause disquiet. If it can cause disquiet, people must be prepared for it. Since screening preschool children raises many issues which are not present in school-age screening, the two populations will be dealt with separately.

Preschool screening: infants and young children

Language milestones have always been incorporated into developmental screening or developmental surveillance since they contain so much information as to the infant's sensory, motor and cognitive abilities. Recently we have seen a change of emphasis in that physicians are being asked to screen for language impairment not only as an indicator of other handicaps (deafness, severe learning impairment) but as a handicapping condition in its own right. The recognition of this claim has caused some paediatricians in the USA to develop their own screening instruments for language (Coplan, 1983; Capute *et al.*, 1986). These seek to extend the developmental screening test most frequently used, the Denver Developmental Scale (Frankenburg *et al.*, 1971) which lacks sufficient early points on language development. In the UK, the hearing screening of all infants by health visitors contributes one essential element to the identification of potential language impairment.

The development of language in infancy and early childhood is now well charted and the factors which contribute to it are also known. Behaviours which indicate that the language acquisition process is taking place can therefore be recorded and used as screening points. Tables 2.2–2.4 show the process in schematic form. Table 2.2 shows how hearing develops from acuity to comprehension in the first year of life. Testing hearing can make use of behavioural responses at, for example, 6 months and 12 months. Table 2.3 shows a similar representation of speech–motor development. Table 2.4 shows the hearing process and the speech–motor process joining to constitute language processes. During the second and third year of life, screening can employ one procedure, e.g. naming, to demonstrate evidence of both speech and hearing ability. The age at which a particular behaviour emerges is left purposely unspecific within a couple of months since too arbitrary a determination is out of keeping with infant variability and can cause anxiety. Comparison of infant developmental scales devised by different authors shows a number of differences within a couple of months on both receptive and expressive language items (Byers Brown, Bendersky and Chapman, 1986; Byers Brown, 1987).

The difficulty in screening infants for possible language delay is to find items which have good predictive validity. Infant development shows both continuities and discontinuities. One skill may precede another but does not necessarily predict another. To say that a child will be delayed in speech because he showed little use of expressive jargon at 11 months is highly unwise. On the other hand an infant who shows no repetitive babble at all during the first year is outside the limit of normal variation.

The developmental outlines tabled (Tables 2.2–2.4) give a broad view of progress in receptive and expressive skills but do not give any information upon interaction, a vital component of language development.

Table 2.2 Hearing acuity – comprehension: Development of communication skills 1

0 (months) 1	2	3	4	5	6	7	8	9	10	11	12
Responds to sounds by startle	Eye blink Eye widening Arousal from sleep Reduction of activity	Responds differently to angry/ friendly, familiar/ unfamiliar voices		Rudimentary head turn to side of sound	Head turn to noise Turns to own name	Localises to side and indirectly below			Responds to 'no'	Localises to side and directly below	
						Turns or smiles to 'Where's Daddy' etc.		Appears to recognise names of self and family		Responds to request plus gesture	

Table 2.3 Speech motor–linguistic activity: Development of communication skills 2

0 (months) 1	2	3	4	5	6	7	8	9	10	11	12
Reflexive crying Vegetative sounds	Reciprocal vocalisation	Cooing Laughter Vocal play	Raspberry (bronx cheer)	Repetitive babbling	Variegated babbling			Expressive jargon		Intentional vocalizing	Sounds and words
	Vowel-type sounds Differentiated crying										

Table 2.4 Receptive and expressive language: Development of communication skills 3

12 (months) 14	16	18	20	22	24	26	28	30	32	34	36
Recognizes familiar rounds *Looks at objects named*		*Recognizes body parts*			*Listens to meaning Points to objects named*			*Obtaining information primarily through language*			
Uses names and function words, e.g. there	Dramatic growth in spoken vocabulary Words with intonation and jargon Initiates communication		Two word utterances		Uses different linguistic elements to vary meaning Word endings Prepositions Word combinations			Sentences expanding in length and complexity			

The only exception is the item 'reciprocal vocalization' at 2–3 months. However, most early developmental and language scales add some items to gauge the extent of a child's general responsiveness and his ability to respond to and to initiate play (peek-a-boo, pat-a-cake). It can be seen that the kind of stimulation in the home would play a decisive part in the child's behaviour in this area.

The object in propagating screening instruments is to allow for the detection of possible abnormality without requiring individual judgement from the person administering the instrument. To invite the administrator to look for mitigating factors or to use his own discretion in the acceptance of a response is to invite disaster. People who carry out screening programmes are not necessarily experts in all aspects of child development. In the UK, the health visitor is an invaluable investigator and one who can carry out a number of procedures which are helpful in the identification of language delay. But the criteria for failure and referral must be clear and unambiguous. Such criteria are easier to establish with regard to hearing and comprehension than they are with regard to speech. Perhaps, if there has to be a partiality, it is much safer to have it this way since hearing and comprehension are so vital for the child's social, cognitive emotional and educational development. Any item on the first year developmental chart for hearing and comprehension (Table 2.2) which the child fails should warrant follow-up. Key screening items can therefore be selected with regard to an unequivocal nature of the behaviour and the ease with which it can be evoked.

A recent report from the US (Kagan, 1988) gives support to the above remarks. Some 4000 children from different regions of the country were administered the Early Learning Milestone Scale or ELM (Coplan, 1983), a brief screening procedure, and their parents responded to a questionnaire. Findings were reviewed for items upon which 400 children provided data. Items were sought which would predict failure for the whole screen. This failure then had to be upheld by failure on a standardised assessment administered by a speech–language pathologist. Two items predicted overall failure from the receptive aspect of the scale. One was failure to orient to a bell within the first year of life. The second was failure to identify common objects described by use ('which one do we play with?') by the end of the second year of life. There were no items from the first or second year of life within the expressive language scale which predicted overall failure. Prediction could only be made with confidence from third year items: uses prepositions, engages in conversation, speaks in two word sentences. This was surprising since the second year items included: use Mama/Dada, uses 4–6 single words; and the first year items included monosyllabic and polysyllabic babble. It should not be inferred that these behaviours are not important or not significant. Taken together with other behaviour, they may indeed reveal that the infant is at risk. However, no one expressive language item should be used as a sole determiner of risk during the first 2 years of life.

Parent report

The five centre study from the US (Kagan, 1988) also yielded information on the relative predictive power of parents when compared with workers administering the screening instrument. Parents were asked whether or not they were concerned about their children's speech or hearing. The sensitivity of parents and the screening tool predicting failure was very much the same. The investigators found that when each was looked at against the standardised assessment, the parents showed a specificity value of 77% and 88% for receptive and expressive aspects respectively and the ELM gave a corresponding specificity of 80% and 85%. Overall, it was found that out of every six children estimated to be at risk for language impairment, five parents were aware of something being wrong. This is for children of 2–36 months of age.

Once more, we must be wary of drawing too strong conclusions. Although the results of the US study suggest that questioning parents would be as valuable as early childhood screening, it does not suggest that parents necessarily volunteer the information. To respond 'Yes' when asked if you are concerned is a different matter from taking your child to the doctor or speech clinic because of this concern. Much of the value of a screening instrument lies in the prompt it gives to primary health workers to direct attention towards significant areas of development. If all children were seen regularly for developmental surveillance during early childhood, and if the relationship between physician and parent were such that easy discussion was a feature of the interview, formal screening would not be necessary. The onus would be upon professionals concerned with speech, language and hearing development to make sure that up-to-date knowledge on important areas was fed through to those responsible for primary health care. Unfortunately, children who fall through surveillance nets are very likely to be disadvantaged children who may be the most at risk.

Speech therapists in the UK are cooperating with paediatricians in reviewing developmental screening policy on a regular basis (Levitt and Muir, 1983; Lindsay, 1984; Health for all Children, 1989). The following points are those which offer the safest guidelines at this stage of our knowledge. Failure indicates the need for follow-up:

0–6 months	Infant responds to sound. Mother expresses no concern about hearing. Infant coos, laughs, reciprocates vocally

6–12 months	Infant localizes to sound. Mother expresses no concern about hearing. Infant vocalises and babbles
12–18 months	Infant locates sound source; carries out one-step commands. Mother expresses no concern about hearing. Infant uses some words spontaneously and correctly.
18–24 months	Infant follows simple instruction without gesture; points to at least one body part when named. Mother expresses no concern about hearing Infant verbally expresses wants; steadily increases number of words used; uses two-word combination around 24 months. Mother expresses no concern about speech

This constitutes the simplest possible screen. Any other signs which place the child at risk (prematurity, genetic hearing loss) should ensure that the child receives a more thorough professional examination at 3-monthly or 6-monthly intervals. The relationship of these early identification procedures to prophylaxis will be discussed in the next chapter.

The single most useful screening procedure between the ages of 24 and 30 months is that focused upon productive vocabulary and the ability to combine words. It has been demonstrated that parents find it easier to recognise the words their children say when shown a vocabulary checklist than when asked to recall them spontaneously during an interview. The procedure advocated by Rescorla (1984) has much to recommend it. The parent is asked to circle, on a comprehensive vocabulary checklist, all the words the child uses spontaneously and then asked to write down examples of sentences, phrases or word combinations. The child fails if he has less than 50 words and no two-word combination.

The British multicentre study (Edwards *et al.*, 1984) made the following comment upon British referral practice for young children. Their children, age range 3–6 years, were referred from a number of agencies, the majority being community based. Less than 10% of the children referred were found to have no speech problems and it was believed that this figure might be lower if all aspects of the communication disorder were taken into account. The report recognises that less obvious difficulties might not have been observed and thus not referred. Nevertheless, the conclusion is that the high validity of the referrals raises questions as to the need for screening instruments. Referrals which are the product of case conferences and informed staff would seem to be both desirable and practicable. Such thinking is in line with current paediatric thinking but may not be acceptable to all. We may expect to see some variability in the extent to which preschool language screening is employed in health districts. It is to be hoped that publication of results will keep us informed as to good practice.

Screening for the school population

As the child approaches school age, screening for language delay or disorders becomes easier in that there are many more markers. Normal 4 year olds converse and narrate by means of intelligible speech. Phonology and grammar have been sufficiently well documented through child language research to generate reliable screening guidelines. It will be for the speech therapy and education services to decide what kind of identification system to put into effect. No quick screen will pick up the subtle problems of comprehension or interaction which indicate language disorders of the semantic–pragmatic type. The quicker the test, the more it tends to focus upon articulation as a criterion. Those responsible may therefore decide that rather than institute a one-off screening procedure, they will invest in teacher-based identification procedures. The ethical considerations still apply. Once a child has been identified as being at risk he must be given diagnostic and remedial services. If these are not available educational authorities will not wish to have possible problems identified. On the other hand without some kind of screening of the school population, the need for services cannot be calculated and the services planned.

The Association For All Speech Impaired Children (AFASIC, 1988) is currently validating an experimental version of its screening test designed for children from 5 to 11 years of age. The test is specifically designed for administration by teachers. It therefore has a dual purpose: the identification of language-impaired children and the education of teachers in this complex subject. The instructions state that the child should be reasonably well known to the teacher before the test is administered. A period of observation prior to administration may be necessary. The reason for these injunctions becomes clear when the test is studied. Information is sought on all major areas pertaining to language disorder, motor, cognitive and play behaviour as well as language measures. A profile is compiled which will then indicate the main areas of deficit and strength. The role of such a test has yet to be explored. It takes time to prepare for and to administer and yet in no way precludes the need for full assessment once the child is identified as at risk. Teachers who lack recourse to specialists in language disorders may find such a profile gives them enough help in working with the child to justify the time spent. Others, who have more ready access to other services may prefer to follow a simple list of questions such as that compiled by Beveridge and Conti-Ramsden (1987). Samples are 'Does the pupil often misunderstand simple instructions?. . . .not seem fully to understand logical correctives?. . . .avoid tasks and situations involving language?' The teacher may then request further investigation or not according to the pattern of response.

Dewart and Summers (1988) have recently constructed a Pragmatics Profile of Early Communication Skills which promises to be a useful addition to our identification procedures. This instrument was developed to extend the range of the clinician's investigations by obtaining information on a number of communicative behaviours in a variety of contexts. Thus the investigator would be able to build up a more realistic picture of the child as a communicator than could be gained from clinic or classroom alone.

A working model

At the present stage of service development in the UK we need to concentrate on the identification of a child's difficulties by those responsible for his care. This point is well argued by Beveridge and Conti-Ramsden in the text just cited. It makes excellent sense for those who provide or witness the main bulk of a child's linguistic experience to be carefully attuned to the way in which he is responding to it. In 1985, the City of Birmingham, UK appointed a teacher to its Visiting Teacher Service to set up a system for helping children with speech and language impairments in mainstream schools. In her description of the programme Locke (1989) defines the initial screen as being the means of bringing the class teacher's attention to any child who is not communicating as often or as effectively as the majority of children in the class. Such a screen should not require extensive explanation, should be quick and easy to administer and should make use of the teacher's everyday observations of the child's language skills. The Birmingham procedure provides for first identification to take place within the first half-term of a child's school enrolment. It is followed by first level intervention by the teacher who uses general strategies suggested by the visiting teacher. A full programme of evaluation, second level intervention and evaluation are developed with guidance lines for referral. Materials are demonstrated and provided by the Visiting Teacher Service.

This kind of programme seems to place identification within the most productive framework. The child has immediate access to support and eventual access to specialist assistance if required. The teacher gains in skill and confidence without having to devote an excessive amount of time to one particular problem. There is no risk of duplicating assessment procedures by instigating a number of specialist referrals in the first instance. Over time, the awareness of language disorders should steadily increase together with awareness of how to ameliorate their effects.

Identification of later language learning difficulties

Language growth represents a slow, gradual continuum of change and modification. During the process there are periods of acceleration and periods where nothing much seems to be happening. These periods may represent reorganisations which will then be followed by further growth. Children will be presented with educational challenges and increased cognitive demands during their school careers. It is likely that some of these demands cannot be met by children whose earlier language abilities appeared adequate. Reasons are indicated in the earlier discussion of maturational lag. Teachers need to be sensitive to the effects of new language demands upon children who were at any time delayed in speech since their time-scale of growth may be different from their peers. They may have longer plateau periods and less acceleration between plateaux. Children who have shown early, slight, motor difficulties in combination with delayed language may break down again at a much later age when demands for writing at speed are made.

Other manifestations of language inadequacy might be unruly and disruptive behaviour in class and lack of participation in group discussions. Children who find that they cannot follow group instructions are likely to react in this way. Children who become aware of differences between their own ability to absorb and generate information through language and those of their peers may become obstreperous or withdrawn. Truanting offers a way out for some and illness for others. There are, of course, other reasons why older children and adolescents start to rebel against their teachers or against the school system in general. Nevertheless, language disability must always be considered when such behaviour follows an early history of speech delay.

The most helpful way in which speech therapists can contribute to the identification of these later difficulties is to ensure that all early problems of spoken language are well documented. Snowling (1985b) observes that speech therapists, working at the interface of medicine and education, in preschool and primary school play a crucial role in the prevention, early detection, assessment and management of children's written language difficulties. She believes that speech therapists should be involved at every stage in identifying, monitoring and, where appropriate, treating the specific educational needs of individuals who, if not in their care, have at some stage passed through it. This belief is underscored in a 1985 text on Children's Written Language Difficulties edited by Snowling (Snowling, 1985a); one contributor, Stackhouse, writes about the relationship between phonetic speech difficulties and subsequent spelling problems. Ideally, speech therapists should keep under review children with reduced phoneme–grapheme correspondence since, although their speech may have improved, they are at risk for spelling problems. The extent to which this can be done will, of course, depend upon the numbers of children involved and the extent of speech therapy provision.

It will be seen that the identification of language disorder, whether latent or present, is a multidisciplinary function. Although the alarm may be given by one person, parent or professional, that alarm will be given much more readily and accurately if a lot of what is known by specialists can be filtered through to those who are in daily contact with the child. Specialist knowledge will itself be increased and buttressed by the feedback received from those whose interest they have succeeded in alerting. Specialists also have a responsibility to see that the child's difficulties and abilities are well documented and that this documentation is available to those who inherit the child as a pupil. The fact that children may receive speech therapy under the auspices of the health service can prevent those in education becoming aware of the child's history. Breakdown can also occur if a child moves into another school district or simply moves from primary to secondary school. Such breakdown can only be prevented by vigilance on the part of everyone involved.

Chapter 3
Prevention*

Summary

This chapter looks again at the factors which may place a child at risk for language disorder, in order to see how their impact can be minimised. It considers the general nature of prevention through public and professional education. Specific reference is made to a number of prophylactic measures which may be advocated. Suggestions for parent guidance are given. Particular attention is paid to the ways in which secondary features of the disorder can be prevented. Examples both of useful books and good practice are given. Speech and language precursors are discussed in some detail in relation both to detection and prevention of abnormality.

The more we know about how language disorders develop the greater becomes our responsibility to try to prevent them. Professional growth may be judged by the way it moves from correction to overall management. There are few speech pathologists who have taken an interest in the general principles of prevention, Michael Marge of the USA being one of the best known (Marge, 1984). Marge distinguishes between primary, secondary and tertiary prevention which we will redefine here.

Primary prevention

This is the elimination or inhibition of the onset or development by altering susceptibility or reducing exposure for susceptible persons. An

*Since this chapter contains many descriptions of mother–child interactions the pronoun 'he' has consistently been used for the child to contrast with 'she' for the mother. The device should be viewed as one chosen to promote clarity and ease of reading rather than indicating gender preference.

example would be the protection from ear infections which might lead to hearing loss and delayed language development.

Secondary prevention

This is early detection which may lead to elimination of the disorder, retardation of its progress and prevention of further complications. Early hearing screening is an instance of this. If a conductive hearing loss were found, the infant could receive medical or surgical treatment to reverse the disease process and language stimulation to promote language learning.

Tertiary prevention

This constitutes the reduction of a disability through the promotion of effective function. Should the infant's hearing loss prove to be irreversible, means to aid residual hearing and to teach language must be put into effect. If successful they should allow the child to benefit from education to the full and to develop socially and emotionally to his full potential.

Speech therapists must be concerned with prophylaxis which can be seen as the taking of an active step towards prevention. They may not be able to shield a child from ear infections but they can see that he is protected from adverse linguistic consequences through efficient hearing testing and language guidance. Some of the means they can employ have already been indicated. For example, one of the major practices of secondary prevention is the mass screening of persons without symptoms.

Language delays and disorders are themselves secondary to biological and environmental conditions. So in considering how we can prevent these delays and disorders, we are faced by a number of factors outside our control. Here we can only hope to intervene effectively at the secondary or tertiary level. There are other conditions where we may hope to prevent the language abnormality from occurring in the first place. The points upon which we can impact to alter factors adverse to language development will be discussed together with the practicalities of prophylaxis. Tertiary prevention will be considered more fully in Chapter 7 since it is part of language intervention.

Public and professional awareness

The first part of any campaign for primary or secondary prevention is the raising of the general consciousness about deleterious practice and how to avoid it. Infants are at biological risk for language disorders as for other developmental problems if they are conceived by sick parents, damaged *in utero*, malnourished, small for dates and pre-term. They are at risk if they are born into poisonous environments and undernourished. All educated people who are able to inform themselves on these points have a duty to campaign on the side of a healthy society. Speech therapists are one of the professional groups which see the consequences to children of any kind of abuse; they will therefore wish to associate themselves with all movements designed to improve infant health and to protect children from the consequences of adult ignorance and shortsightedness. Their direct responsibilities are for communication and language.

One of the authors of this text (BBB) took part in an exercise in New Jersey (USA) designed to promote an efficient, coordinated scheme through which to identify infants and young children who were at risk for or suffering from communication disorders. Preliminary investigation suggested that there were a number of systems of services in which such children could be involved. These service systems comprised hospital or diagnostic centre, community clinic, and maternal and child health programmes. The children could also be identified through one of several parallel child-care systems including state efforts to implement the Education for All Handicapped Children Act, State Developmental Disabilities Programs, Head Start and Early Intervention Services either home or centre based. There were also a number of facilities developed by voluntary health agencies and private practitioners in paediatrics, audiology, psychology and speech–language pathology. There seemed little point in attempting to add to these facilities. The research team therefore determined to promote, augment and seek to coordinate those service systems which were already in use. Through careful study of the way in which the systems were being used, we would hope to find out what lay behind the general complaint that children were not being referred early enough to benefit fully from speech, language and hearing services.

Underlying the research team's efforts was the rationale that since no one single profession is responsible for all aspects of care, successful management must involve the coordination of different aspects of professional responsibility. Thus, once more we were drawn to look at the systems within which professionals worked. Attention was also directed towards parent and public education since this creates the climate within which systems of care may flourish. The aims of the project were as follows:

- To improve the general level of public and professional awareness.
- To improve the skills of those involved in primary identification.
- To offer more resources to those concerned with diagnosis and management.
- To identify specific weaknesses in the identification and referral systems.

All these points are directly concerned with prevention, primary, secondary and tertiary.

The project

The target population was children aged 0–4 in a four-county area of New Jersey. The research team first announced its intention to promote better identification of children at risk for communication disorders through newspaper and state professional bulletins, radio and television pro-grammes. It invited cooperation and appealed for information on existing facilities. Special meetings were held with the New Jersey Speech and Hearing Association and with other organisations serving handicapped children. There was also full discussion with the New Jersey State Department of Health followed by cooperative investigation carried out jointly by the research team and by those in charge of the Newborn Hearing Program for High Risk Infants. As a result, two major studies were mounted by the research team which was based in the Department of Pediatrics of the State medical school. The first study examined the Newborn Screening Program which had reported a compliance rate of only 17%. It was considered that if children known to be at risk attracted such a poor screening response, there would be little point in attempting to develop further programmes until the reasons were known.

Table 3.1 shows the deficiencies revealed and the remedies proposed. The deficiencies arose mainly from lack of communication between the various groups, administrative, professional and parental, which were involved. However, there was a general lack of faith in the screening process which needed to be tackled directly. The remedies proved to be effective as was indicated by a considerable increase in the compliance rate at the end of the next year. Regular revision of the programme should ensure that this continues and improves still further.

The second study was undertaken to establish the identity of those professionals who assessed young children for communication disorders. Professionals in the USA command a very wide range of employers when compared with the UK where the NHS is the major employer, at least of

Table 3.1 Investigation of Newborn Hearing program for High Risk Infants (Study 1)

Deficiencies revealed	Remedies initiated
Parents inadequately informed regarding:	Parent education
1. Reasons for child's registration	Public and professional information campaign
2. Procedures	Revised criteria for inclusion
3. Financial assistance	Additional subsidised assessment centres
Physicians not convinced regarding:	Screening training
1. Value of programme	Entire programme revised by State
2. Reasons for inclusion	Department of Health
3. Results of own screening	
4. Effectiveness of early diagnosis	

speech therapists. Private practice was particularly prosperous in New Jersey. Table 3.2 shows the deficiencies revealed and remedies initiated. A conspicuous finding was the dearth of assessment instruments available for very young children as distinct from those of between 2;6 and 4 years of age. From this study we were able to calculate the number of children in different age groups who reached the assessors. We learned more about referral routes and the conditions most likely to prompt referrals. As a consequence we were able to decide where to concentrate our attack in the attempt to improve identification. The establishment of a baseline number of referrals for the different ages meant that we were also able to measure our own efforts by the subsequent increase in numbers. These efforts included a number of training sessions for paediatricians and nurses together with presentations at professional conferences and a variety of medical and educational centres.

Table 3.2 Identification of assessors in early child communication (Study 2)

Deficiencies revealed	Remedies initiated
1. Delay in referral	Continuing education for primary care
2. Delay in assessment after referral	personnel and for those who assess
3. Inadequate assessment instruments	Promotion of new techniques
4. Inappropriate assessment instruments	Propagation of research findings on
5. Lack of parental interest	development of communication skills
6. Lack of services for 0–2 year olds	Parent education
	New sites for screening and assessment
	Revision of assessment tools
	Research into communicative behaviour of
	0–2 year olds

The research team carried out its own studies into early communication development and as a result suggested a number of items which were then incorporated into both screening and assessment procedures. Language items were added to the hearing items which constituted the main follow-up procedure in communication screening for infants at risk due to prematurity or genetic factors. The overall result was to reduce the waiting time between first identification and subsequent assessment for all children but particularly for the younger ones and considerably to increase the number of appropriate referrals. Once more, it is considered that the procedures should continue to promote better practice.

It became apparent during the studies described above, that screening programmes will deteriorate unless very serious efforts are made to maintain them. Table 3.3 indicates some of the factors leading to deterioration in some of the New Jersey programmes. They have their counterpart elsewhere. Indeed, the point of describing the New Jersey

Table 3.3 Conditions and circumstances leading to deterioration of screening programmes

Conditions	Causes	Remedies initiated
Time pressure	Over scheduling Emergencies Number and variety of tasks to be accomplished Financial profit	Task analysis Elimination of redundant and unnecessary procedures Assistance from research personnel in conducting screening
Lack of knowledge	Training in procedures only without teaching of principles and background Complex nature of communicative development	Regular demonstration and discussion of cases In-service training Distribution of reading material Research team available for reference
Staff change	Unsatisfactory conditions Inadequate remuneration Natural wastage	Beyond the efforts of research staff except as above to improve morale
Lack of feedback	Parents fail to follow through Screening personnel not informed of results of assessment	Continuous and sustained effort to improve flow of information Parent interviews Professional conferences Preparation of suitable forms of exchange of information
Low morale	Associated with all the factors recorded above	All measures indicated above plus expression of appreciation

Some of the remedies put into effect by research staff could not be maintained beyond the life of the project. Others were incorporated into the system and continue to be effective. A main contribution of the research was to indicate the extent to which a system is vulnerable to breakdown and to recommend review procedures.

project is to draw attention to the counterparts which exist in other countries. Systems of health care may differ but the needs and behaviour of people working in them will be the same. The success of the research project was, of course, very much due to the funds it had available to produce materials and to help mount activities. Nevertheless, the most important factor was almost certainly staff enthusiasm and time spent with the primary care personnel. When a research staff member was present, identification of communication problems became a focus of interest. Once she left, time became swallowed up by other things. The moral is very clear. We cannot mount programmes to identify and to prevent conditions occurring unless there are funds to maintain them and unless there are people who have a major interest and continuing investment in them. Another point to be made is that speech therapists must find ways of having an impact upon the systems controlling health care and education if prophylactic measures are to be developed.

Prevention–detection

If early detection of language delay is to be a serious venture, allies must be sought among those professionals involved in developmental surveillance: the family doctor, the paediatrician, the health visitor and community nurse. In the UK, the health visitor has long been trained in hearing screening, among other activities. She is consequently in a very good position to carry out any other procedures related to communication development. Ward (1984) describes a study in which health visitors were chosen to administer questionnaires about auditory behaviour because parents were familiar with their interest in hearing and would not become anxious when questioned by them.

The success of health visitors in making appropriate referrals to the speech therapist has already been indicated in this text. An essential part of any in-service programme through which to train health visitors would be the demonstration of early delays and deviations and possible outcomes. When referrals are made, full information on the results of the assessment should be fed back as speedily as possible. When this is not done, enthusiasm wanes and potential skills are wasted. Since the health visitor is likely to be in demand for a number of important duties, it is obviously essential not to add to her activities without giving her the job satisfaction to which she is entitled.

Screening and first identification procedures should be brief and easy to administer as has been emphasised in Chapter 2. Nevertheless, there are minimum standards which must be met. An attempt was made in New Jersey to enlist the aid of community nurses in Well Baby clinics and this immediately threw up the difficulty inherent in almost every baby clinic site. Some of the places in which the nurses worked were extremely noisy and crowded, and there was almost invariably pressure of time. In addition to their own busy schedules, the nurses had to consider mothers with a number of fretful small children, all anxious to get home. There was scarcely ever a refusal to cooperate, only an understandable temptation to put on one side any matters which were not causing anxiety. Professionals are continually forced to compromise between their own interests and those of the parents, but there are many instances where compromise is not possible. It is far better that the procedures should not be attempted at all and this fact recorded in the case history than that the procedure should be carried out too cursorily with the risk of an inaccurate result.

The preventive aspect of early identification is its strongest weapon and this should always be fully explained. One screening programme which was carried out among a largely middle-class professional White population was ill received because the parents perceived it as an assessment procedure and considered that it did not do justice to their children's abilities. If screening is to be used continually as a preventive measure, we cannot afford to have the procedures fall into disrepute. As a means of educating public opinion, it may not be the best way to proceed. If the intention is to locate children who are at risk for a condition known to be prevalent and punitive, general screening may well be advocated. The important thing is to use this vehicle, as all others, with judgement and in a spirit of enthusiastic realism.

As the child enters into a larger world, he has more opportunity both to practice language skills and to reveal language deficiencies. Instead of the mother and health care professionals being the only judges of the child's attainment, there are likely to be nursery teachers, nursery aides, play group managers, day care centre staff and others who have the opportunity to look at an individual child in the company of his peers. Helping a non-verbal child to experience and enjoy language and to try to communicate are very reasonable goals within small social groups. Where the number of children is large and the number of adults small, no great benefits can be expected. However, even in these cases identification of communication delays is possible, particularly when there is good working contact with the speech therapy service. Where identification is possible, some prophylactic measures may be applied.

A child's differing environment may have a role to play in altering susceptibility. For example, if a child is born into a family where there is a tendency towards delayed language, his parents may request his early admission to a nursery which offers more stimulating play and musical materials than the home can provide. The child may also receive more communicative challenge. Conversely, nursery staff may observe that a child becomes more confused and tired than his peers when verbally stimulated. They may suggest that the child spends more time with a single care-giver who can give him more individual guidance until his attention and listening skills improve.

Young children joining nursery or play groups for the first time become prone to infections. If a child has already experienced a number of episodes of otitis media in infancy he is at increased risk for further episodes in childhood. Nursery staff may be very helpful in noting a child's response to sounds and advising his parents of the need to seek medical opinion.

Children who lack communicative opportunity or communicative effort may benefit considerably from an extension of their environment. If they have to communicate in order to satisfy needs or gratify wishes, they will try to do so. Observant adults may note whether the attempts to communicate increase the child's skills or cause him distress. They can give help, or withold it, in the light of their judgement. Thus a new situation is one which provides opportunity to detect, support, report and possibly teach necessary skills.

Prevention--information

To give people useful information is not necessarily to make them act more wisely but it does give them the opportunity. Since so much of what we know about good language development technique has come from our observation of parents, it is only right that we feed back to parents the results of our observations. Outstandingly, we have learned that no one theory of language development based upon formal linguistic studies or single cognitive or perceptual systems can suffice to explain language development (Trevarthen, Murray and Hubley, 1981): 'Infants communicate by using all their faculties in sensitive dependence on both the human and the practical, useable environment.' The infant, although seemingly highly dependent upon his mother for language nourishment, has been shown to be capable of exerting considerable control, even in very early exchanges. His gradual mastery of language is part of a dynamic, interactive process in which his behaviour stimulates the mother towards skilful support and education (see Lewis and Freedle, 1973; Lewis, 1977; Trevarthen, Murray and Hubley, 1981; Trevarthen and Marwick, 1986).

Trevarthen and Marwick (1986) point out that the intrinsic motivation of the expressive and receptive processes in the child's mind is so strong that it is unlikely that his behaviour will simply reflect the frequency of occurrence of particular items in the mother's activity. Parents then should be reassured that they are not responsible for teaching the child to talk by following any particular method. Nor are they responsible for any slowness he may show in talking simply because they have failed to indulge in any one speech-oriented activity during the early months of life. They will only be responsible if they fail to supply a happy relationship for the baby with a person easily and frequently available to him.

Some of the effects of our early discoveries on the importance of early language development may have been to over-emphasise the role of 'mother-talk' simply as talk. Although mothers who are naturally chatty and expressive may greatly enjoy talking to their very young babies, others may not find it so easy. So the less exuberant mothers will read with relief that the quality of their responses, the way in which they react by smiling, touching and directing the infant's attention to objects of interest will serve the infant just as well. He does need to learn that he can have an effect upon his environment, that communicative effort brings rewards and that sustained response to visual and auditory experiences is enjoyable. The first two of these he can only learn through adult help. The third he will learn if adults refrain from interfering with his enjoyment by offering competing stimuli. At a somewhat later stage they will help by providing materials calculated to hold his interest and showing him how to attend to them.

Mother—child talk

As babies grow into toddlers and children, their mothers change the way in which they speak to them. The changes reflect the mother's recognition of her child's developing understanding of language and then of his attempts to speak. The earliest speech from mothers to babies uses a wide range of intonation and is emotional in content. It uses rhetorical questions and attributes moods and feelings to the baby. The baby himself and his state and features constitute the dominant theme and the tone is one of great warmth. As the baby grows older, the content of the mother's speech changes to reflect and extend his interest in his environment. Comments on objects and activities which are immediately apparent take the place of comments on the child's moods and feelings. These changes in mother-talk occur when the baby is around 3—4 months old. During the first few months parents start to be aware of the infant's attention to speech and perceive the beginning of comprehension or word recognition. This leads them to use more naming and repetition.

As the infant starts to produce words, the mother responds in such a way as to affirm his attempts and encourage him to continue. His parents perceive the child's use of words as a further sign of his understanding of language and so continue to use language as a means, not only of stimulating and encouraging him but of controlling his behaviour. The Bristol study (Wells, 1985) showed that parents relied upon language to control children as young as 15 months. The directives tended to be short and simple but used the normal adult grammer. The use of speech for control purposes is, of course, unlikely to be effective unless supported by physical action. Unless a child associates the removal of an object with an injunction against banging it, kicking it, throwing it down etc., then spoken injunctions are unlikely to restrain him. This simple example immediately throws up the impossibility of disassociating spoken language from all the complexities of the child—mother relationship and of its individual nature.

Lieven (1982) points out the number of processes that are involved in children talking in a real-world situation. Her paper goes on to discuss the complex ways in which a child's progress in speech impinges upon factors of general learning and is affected by his social world:

> Whenever a child says something all of the following factors will be involved: contextual priming, memory, current strategies for producing utterances, and the conventions and attitudes which govern talk in the world in which the child lives.

Lieven's paper moves from discussing the characteristics of speech to children to emphasise the importance of individual variation. Her main tenet is that by separating the study of child language into areas such as 'cognitive underpinning', 'input' and 'generation of formal linguistic rules' we distort the object of study.

Crystal (1986), in a text for parents, illustrates most aptly how research into child language can inform lay people. Teachers and clinicians who take unto themselves the task of advising parents have to try to retain and abstract what is 'good practice' from the revised ideas and current enthusiasms of the research field. At the present time (Summer 1988) the following points may be made when giving instruction to caregivers on how to assist language development in very young children. They have already been well tested and are likely to be durable. The age limits are, of course, approximations.

The first 3 months

Talk to your baby during the periods of physical caring and cuddling. Use natural warm loving tones, playful tones, crooning as your feelings dictate. Respond to your baby's cooing sounds by imitating him or by showing pleasure, smiling and listening. Encourage his sound play by imitating his sounds and adding a few variations of your own. Comment on his looks and behaviour and interpret them aloud.

From 3 to 6 months

Look for different responses to angry and soothing, familiar and unfamiliar voices. Vary the volume and tones of your voice in order to draw your baby's attention to different objects. Make use of all caring routines like bathing and nappy changing to tell your baby what is going on. Enjoy the responses, smiling, vocalising. Start simple play routines using parts of the body ('This little piggy went to market', 'Walkie round the garden, like a Teddy Bear' etc.). Start showing simple outline picture books and telling about what you see.

From 6 to 9 months

Draw baby's attention to common household sounds and voices. Ask questions like 'Where's daddy?' Where's pussy?' and supply answers 'Here he is'. Play 'Peekaboo'. Use books and toys to interest the baby in names: 'Here's a big car', 'Look at the funny dog'. Respond to baby's communicative signals, shrieks, pointing, bouncing up and down and interpret the signals in words 'You want your milk?', 'You don't like that hat' 'Yes, we're going to go out now'. He may like to joggle about while you sing.

From 9 to 12 months

Talk about things that are happening every day. Use simple, clear speech and make use of routines in order to establish the connection between language and events. Follow the infant's lead. If he indicates something, talk about that. If he is not interested in a book or toy, don't push it but talk about something else. Listen to his attempts to speak and try to interpret them within the context of what you are both doing. Encourage and enjoy but don't demand imitation of your speech. Give the infant plenty of time to respond to your speech and don't carry on a continuous monologue. He will have his own thoughts.

The overall theme is that of interaction and communication. During the first year the mother introduces the baby to ways in which he can participate in and then control his environment. She does this from a basis of consistent, loving nurture. Prevention of delay at this level lies in the promotion of interaction, not the specific reinforcement of training of any single prespeech skill. By the end of the first year the infant should be capable of recognising words and phrases that reoccur frequently in his daily life. His own utterances may be of a number of types and this will affect the way in which his parents attempt to encourage him. First, they will adapt their language to the level at which they perceive the child comprehends. Secondly they will respond to the kind of utterance the child uses.

The process of language discovery by the child, assisted by the parent, is both highly pleasurable and non-didactic. The process is not one which proceeds through attention to language rules but through the pleasure of each participant in the behaviour of the other. Those who really enjoy the discovery of language can use it to build skills and interests which will be of permanent benefit to the child. The extension of the process in this way is beautifully illustrated in Dorothy Butler's delightful treatise *Babies need Books* (Butler, 1988). Butler starts by attempting to interest babies in books when they are a few months old. A book that has bright, simple outline on a white page will attract the baby's attention if he is shown it at a propitious time, i.e. when alert but not tired, fretful, hungry or wet. Butler points out that the business of holding the baby and directing his attention to the picture is pleasurable for both parties so the experience will not be a total loss, even if the child responds little. Butler develops her theme by making very practical, concrete suggestions as to the best books to use at different ages.

Such a practice as regular reading to the child is one that can be thoroughly recommended to all parents but it does need to be practically followed up. If people are not used to having books around the home, they will need to be told what to find and how to find it. They will need directing towards infant book and toy libraries and then towards public libraries. It must be explained to parents who are not themselves readers that books offer the infant a much richer experience than does the over-stimulating television screen. This may have a place later on but not for the very young child who needs to identify a few things over and over again in circumstances of quiet caring. As parents start to use simple books they will become more interested in seeking out others. The television screen does not allow selection or participation in this way.

The early use of books to give pleasure and stimulate interest in language is a far cry from the techniques which are designed to turn infants into prodigies. These have no place in this text. An infant who has learnt early in life that books are attractive objects will have a constant source of language nourishment. Not only his parents but all visiting adults may be pressed into reading to him or talking about pictures. He will soon learn to name the pictures and memorise short passages and so can display his own skill in 'reading aloud'. This will naturally encourage him to master reading and his developing language skills will increase the likelihood of his doing so.

Sharing a book with a young child is also very enjoyable for the adult. Not only does it provide a less exhausting form of entertainment than most but it allows for early conversation which a lack of intelligibility on the one side and resourcefulness on the other might otherwise preclude. If two people are looking at a picture and one makes some kind of noise, it is easy for the other to say 'Yes, it is a dog, a big black dog' etc. This 'shared focus' is one of the aspects of motherese and one which has led to its promotion as a teaching technique. (See also Whitehurst *et al.* (1988) on accelerating language development through picture book reading.)

Prevention–intervention

The first year

Interest in associating mother-talk with the earliest stages of the mother–child relationship is now sufficiently strong to prompt early intervention. An example can be found in Boston, USA where a number of steps were taken to help mothers from disadvantaged and disturbed backgrounds in interacting with their babies. The babies were born to mothers who were not prepared for them and did not know how to manage them. Some were teenagers, many were single parents, many had histories of disturbed or antisocial behaviour. It was hoped that by promoting the skills of parenting, professionals might be able to encourage a more hopeful and positive outlook in the mothers. The speech–language pathologist's contribution to the programme was presented at the American Speech–Language–Hearing Association convention (Proctor, 1982). The mothers were shown how to incorporate loving, warm-toned speech into their caring routines. Wide-ranging intonation, cooing, singing and other gentle, expressive vocalisations were used by the speech–language pathologists and the mothers were asked to imitate. The object was to start a communicative, loving interaction through voice which could be easily perpetuated and developed as the baby responded.

The idea is certainly an appealing one but it needs to be propagated with great care. If mothers are feeling angry, bewildered, frightened or helpless, the attempt to teach them to speak in warm soothing tones will be at best useless and at worst harmful. The infant may very well be frightened and confused by the mixed messages coming from sentimental words with an underlay of hostility and soothing tones with an edge of fear. Counselling and practical help with social needs and personal problems must precede or at least accompany guidance in how to change language behaviour.

There are prophylactic measures to help unresponsive babies and those at risk for language delay which are simply attempts to give normal experience in a heightened way. Such measures may be found in a number of texts on early communication (e.g. Coupe and Goldbart, 1987; Warner, 1987). When the infant is at risk for profound handicap, early efforts may be concentrated on showing him how he can affect his environment. Parents and caregivers are advised how to make their responses contingent upon the infant's attempts to move, vocalise or look. Not only does the infant gain pleasure from the response but he starts to realise that activity is productive. He learns that what he does makes a difference to what happens to him. In order to increase an infant's awareness of the importance of language, we must help him first to make sense of what he hears.

Auditory stimulation

All babies benefit from help in listening selectively to environmental sounds since these are now so many and varied that their total impact can be overwhelming. Parents may need guidance with babies who are unresponsive to sound and babies who are distressed by sound since these may indicate real problems in auditory perception and processing as well as in acuity. Demonstration should be given of how to attract the infant's interest towards a soundmaker by first making it a focus of visual interest. When the noise is produced, the object is well in view and the noise can be repeated. Many parents make the mistake of trying to test a child's reactions to sound by making noises behind his back or when he is engrossed in some activity. Such tactics may achieve a once only response if the sound is loud but they are not part of auditory training. The training consists of building up associations between sounds and objects and activities. If the infant is unresponsive, the mother may be shown how to heighten interest by using an attractive toy with a squeaker, or by rattling a brightly coloured box with something inside, opening the box, taking the object out, putting it back and rattling it again. Caregivers should be advised to show infants the sources of sound by carrying them to the window when the cars are hooting, tracking down the telephone when it rings, listening as well as looking when the television is turned on. Then the range of sounds should be increased: the sound of paper being torn or crumpled, sugar being sifted, tea being stirred.

Children who are not able to attach meaning to sounds will start to ignore them. In some cases this can lead to profound inhibition and withdrawal (Ward, 1984). If this seems to be the case, carefully graded auditory stimulation should be given by professionals in the parents' presence to make sure that everyone knows the limit of the child's tolerance. If babies show excessive sensitivity to sounds, parents should be encouraged to persist in reducing fear. When household objects are being used which generate sudden noise (and there are a great many of these), the infant should, where possible, be prepared. The object should be within his sight and the parent should say 'Here it is, it's going to make a noise' then generate the noise for a short while and then switch the machine off and comment again. The object with all controlled auditory stimulation is to keep the child aware of sounds as being potentially meaningful without letting him become overwhelmed and distressed by them. The stimulation may thus involve capitalising upon the normal and inevitable noises of the household. It should also include quiet times when small sounds and quiet music may be enjoyed and books may be read.

Sound production

As well as responding to environmental sounds and to the speech of others, the infant needs to enjoy the sounds he can produce himself. He first learns the effect of his sounds on others by parental response to his crying. If he is to move on to master the complexities of a speech—sound system as a vehicle for communication, he must get some satisfaction from his early attempts. He is able to demonstrate to others that he is physically capable of generating streams of sound well before he is expected to use speech. If he fails to demonstrate this, there will be concern about his potential for spoken language. Thus the babbling period of babyhood is extremely important because the infant receives pleasure and reinforcement in speech—sound production and the parents are reassured about his speech productive ability. The phenomenon of babbling will therefore be considered in some detail.

Babbling

A relationship has long been posited between the babble sounds which infants make and the words which they subsequently speak. This putative relationship has been explored by different groups of professionals including those interested in a systematic phonology (Locke, 1983), those interested in the manner in which learning operates upon sound production (Mowrer, 1952; Winitz, 1969) and those concerned with abnormalities of utterance as a means of identifying handicap (Rutter,

Bartak and Newman, 1971; Byers Brown, Bendersky and Chapman, 1986; Rutter, 1987). Rutter has recently drawn attention to babbling as a significant factor in language disorder by including it in his guidelines for the identification of such disorders (Rutter, 1987):

> A disorder may be suspected . . . . if babble has been reduced or unusual in quality . . .

The identification of such babble is, however, no simple matter. Many studies of babbling which is abnormal have been carried out from recordings of infants known to be at risk (Oller, 1980; Grunwell and Russell, 1987). Moreover the recordings must in some cases be subjected to instrumental analysis before the normality or abnormality of the babbling can be determined. This is a far cry from requiring parents to identify 'unusual' babble patterns in their own homes. Byers Brown, Bendersky and Chapman (1986) demonstrated that medical personnel can be trained to distinguish between different kinds of babbling activity and thereby to gain some estimate of the infant's speech–sound age. To do this, though, demands both time and practice. Information about the quality of infant babble is likely to be unreliable therefore. However, information about the timing may be more useful.

Babbling is primarily associated with movement. Kent (1984) suggests that reduplicated babbling is not a limited phonological process but rather a developmental process in which cyclicity is used to motor advantage. This places babbling within a developmental framework in which language and a motor system co-emerge. Stark (1981) previously pointed out that babbling first occurs in the context of playing with objects rather than when interacting with another person. Van der Stelt and Koopmans van Beinum (1986) discussed the significance of babbling within a hierarchical order of motor functioning. If the late babble is one of a series of late emerging motor functions it obviously prompts investigation as part of those functions. Speech therapists are familiar with the lack of babbling reported not only by parents of cerebral palsied children but also by parents of children who turn out to be severely apraxic. In the case of cerebral palsy, work is started with babies as part of a whole neurodevelopmental therapy. Oral movements are stimulated by tactile and kinaesthetic means to promote a number of activities: feeding, kissing, babbling and speech.

Babbling has been a feature of other developmental therapies but here its role is less clear. Certainly it provides a highly pleasurable activity for child and therapist, if the child is very young and the therapist very enthusiastic. Recent research into the number of different strategies used by early speakers suggests that it may not always be the best procedure. Apraxic children have not necessarily been able to bridge the gap between babbling movements and the organized sequence required for speech.

When infants are reported to lack variety in their speech—sound production and to be delayed in gross and fine motor skills, these functions may certainly be stimulated and encouraged together. Rhythmic sound play, singing and clapping games, action games with the child supplying a sound at the end of the sequence are all useful and pleasurable ways of helping movement. They heighten the excitement and thence the activity level which may enable the child to be more productive. However, it may still be important to encourage the use of a communicative strategy consisting of vowels only. If the parent responds to such signals, the child feels success. Moreover, the child may receive the linguistic advantages of contingent maternal speech, shared topic, extension etc. without excessive demands being placed upon his motor skills.

Babbling has been shown to have a place in the assessment of emerging language as a feature of cognition and, conversely, as a feature of cognitive delay and autism. The babbling itself does not demand intervention though it may point the way to other forms of intervention (Wetherby *et al.*, 1986; Del Priore, Valance and Day, 1987). Babbling is also of major interest to phonologists who look to it for first evidence of systematic sound production as a forerunner to phonology. Locke (1983, 1986) has reviewed this subject extensively. Failure to develop a systematic phonology cannot be prevented, however, by intervention at the babbling stage. We might possibly be able to expand the infant's babbling repertoire, if his family tendencies were suggestive of phonological disability. But the phonology could only be developed as words were acquired, which involves another organisational level.

In summary, babbling shows evidence of motor coordination and subsequently of auditory and cognitive alertness. Its absence attracts attention to those areas. Encouraging babbling will not work any miracles but it may give the infant a little push along the developmental path. Any increase of skill opens up possibilities. It indicates responsiveness and evidence of ability to learn. When children are developmentally delayed, all such evidence is important. It will be significant whether the increase in babbling comes about as the result of promoting another type of activity (crawling, object play) or as the result of auditory and linguistic stimulation and interaction.

Speech therapists tend to believe that there is a strong association between lack of babble and subsequent speech disorders. However, as has been pointed out previously, speech therapists have access to a special sample only. There is some research support for the contention that all normal infants babble at some point (van der Stelt and Koopmans van Beinum, 1986). They also coo, laugh, vocalise to smiling adults, use vowel glides and indicate communicative intent. While babble is likely to continue to attract the research field, it should not completely dominate the prophylactic one. Mothers have been known to become very anxious as to whether or not their babies are babbling 'properly.' This does no good to them or to their relationship with their infant. If babies are to be stimulated to babble as part of a guidance programme, it must be done in a relaxed and happy manner.

Babbling stimulation

A vital component of any stimulation programme is knowing when to stimulate. Since the generation of a babble chain demands coordinated activity of breathing, vocalisation and movement of the articulators, it cannot be expected from a very immature mechanism. The literature does not yield cases of repetitive babbling during the first 2 months of life, even in the most advanced babies. We must therefore assume that a number of other activities must take place first. This is why the emphasis in neurodevelopmental therapy is upon a gradual progression from one skill to another. The time to stimulate babbling occurs after the oral reflexes of rooting, sucking and biting have started to wane. The tongue is thus more capable of moving independently. The infant's respiratory health must be such that he is not struggling for breath or breathing so quickly and shallowly that a string of babble sounds cannot be supported. Once an infant has achieved such a string of sounds, he will essay another, even if he has quite severe respiratory congestion. Noisy breathing sounds distressing but does not necessarily prevent babble from emerging. Nevertheless, it is unwise to use tactile and kinaesthetic stimulation in such cases. The adult should rely upon auditory stimulation and smiling, enthusiastic response. If the babble chains occur when the infant is apart from the adult, he should not be interrupted.

Mothers may be encouraged by experienced speech therapists to move the baby's lips and jaw while he is vocalising in order to give him the sensation of what normal movement is like. When such training is given, it is generally in conjunction with a programme of physical therapy. Such training must only take place with careful demonstration and with reference to the one child. If general advice is given, it is wisest to restrict it to such measures as the following:

● Extend the infant's overall desire to move by placing attractive objects so as to encourage head turning, rolling and general pursuit.
● Promote hand and hand-to-mouth activities by giving the infant different objects to hold and to take to his mouth; objects should be such that they cannot be drawn in and swallowed.
● Use sound play with the infant, either by initiating it during phases of lively interaction or by echoing his brief babble attempts.
● Extend the range of babble sounds, e.g. after a number of 'dadada' chains, try 'bababa', use repetitive CV chains until the range is extended and then use combinations 'dadaba' 'bagaga'; vary the stress and volume.

● As babble appears, stimulate general listening skills so that the auditory—motor loop may be strengthened; try to incorporate turntaking into babble practice.

● The final injunction is more difficult to convey. Briefly it is 'do not confuse a thinking baby'. In babbling, as in all skills, the baby may start coming to certain conclusions. He may like the sound he has just made and want to try it again, or he may have made some discovery from it which prompts him to try something else. Everyone concerned with the child should try to understand his own temperament and way of going about things.

Sound imitation

There is general agreement that some children are better mimics or natural imitators than others and this skill is almost certainly helpful in acquiring phonological patterns. The point became masked early in the study of child language acquisition because it was important to establish that language was not learned by imitation but by making deductions from available data. While we do not learn language through imitation, spoken language is facilitated by practice and here imitation has a role to play. Imitation and role learning can improve phonological memory. Thus, repetition of sound patterns, rhymes and even nonsense words may assist the young child to memorise sound sequences at a later stage. Short-term phonological memory is suggested, in a recent research study (Gathercole and Baddeley, 1989), as being associated with development of vocabulary. We are therefore justified in advising mothers to teach children new words through imitation and before this stage to encourage imitation and mimicry of sound patterns. Both immediate and delayed repetition may be employed. While language-delayed children may be slow to acquire words because they lack the overall matrix to support them, others may be slow because of poor phonological skills associated with inability to repeat. Repetition practice at an early age is only likely to do harm if carried out over zealously and humourlessly. Otherwise it may well be generally useful.

Individual variation

By the end of the first year, the infant is already starting to show some individual characteristics or stylistic preferences in speech. This appears to reflect his own disposition rather than that of his family since different siblings show different preferences. Byers Brown and Lewis (1984; Byers Brown, 1988) looked at 50 one year olds (25 male and 25 female) and found the following: during 25 minutes of child—mother interaction the infant's number of utterances ranged from 99 to 1. As well as showing great variation in quantity, there was variation in kind. The most prolific speakers used both variegated and non-variegated babble, vowels with intonation (melodic cadences), vowels in a sequence with or without glottal stop, vocables and words. A positive correlation was found between an overall factor of productive language range and a factor of productive language competence at 2 years of age. This competence factor was derived from the number of connected utterances used by the child, the mean length of these utterances and the ability to use speech to ask questions, generate information and maintain sociability. The authors concluded that the ability to generate a range of utterances at 1 year was a good predictive sign.

A second group of children showed preference for vowel use and relied strongly on the vowel sequence for communication. There was no overall indication to suggest that their language was delayed at 2 years. Some were advanced, some average, some below average. The authors suggested that this vowel preference was a strategy which might be adopted by the less motorically advanced children in that it maintained communication without demanding fine motor control. The vowel sequences /uh uh uh uh/ were often used with a degree of urgency which demanded a communicative response. Children who used babble and melodic cadence might use them with or without seeming to desire the attention of the mother. These strategies were both expressive of mood and useful in conveying mood and information (not always interpretable by the adult!). The vowel sequence was only used communicatively and thus could be associated with children who were not highly expressive overall.

A third group of 1 year olds tended to rely upon simple consonant–vowel combinations uttered somewhat explosively – 'da'. They did not generate long utterances. A positive correlation was found between this factor of consonant use and a factor of unintelligible (or inadequate) utterance at 2 years. A negative correlation was found between the factor of consonant use and the factor of productive language competence at 2 years. The authors suggested that the consonant use strategy was one employed by the least able communicators, or perhaps by those least interested in communication.

Implications for prevention

Since the children taking part in the above study were only recorded with their mothers at 1 year and then at 2 years, it is not possible to speak about the influence either of the mother's speech or of her behaviour. What the study does illustrate is the strategic choice available and the possibilities of a mismatch of style and temperament between mother and child. Some mothers were equally responsive to a 1 year old using grunts, points and vowel sequences as to the 2 year old using words. One could opine that this responsiveness was a factor in the child's progress. Other mothers noticeably communicated much less with their 1 year olds than with their 2 year olds. Where the child was strongly expressive and communicative himself, this did not seem to deter him. The combination of an uncommunicative, unexpressive child and an unresponsive mother, though very understandable, was not very propitious.

We can only speculate on the possible effects on interaction when the child is inexpressive and uncommunicative and the mother is highly expressive. In one mother–child dyad observed by Byers Brown and Lewis, the mother talked continuously to her unresponsive, inattentive 1 year old. He produced his only continuous utterance, a repetitive babble chain, while his mother was briefly out of the room. At 2 years of age the child was non-communicative and the mother unable to engage him. Whose behaviour was the most responsible? Just as such paediatricians as Brazelton gave mothers enormous relief by telling them that they had difficult babies, or that they would have done a fine job with a baby of a different temperament, so speech therapists may make the same kind of observations to mothers of speech-delayed children. The mother, as the more skilled partner, has the onus on her to promote language development in the child. However, some mothers have a much easier time than others.

We must await the completion of longitudinal studies by such workers as Bates and Lieven before we can say much more about the range of individual variation and different linguistic characteristics of the mother–child dyad. The wisest course is to emphasise that the range of infant variation exists in all information aimed at promoting good, early language development. When recommending texts to mothers who want to know more about the process, choose those in which information is blended with humour and affection (Crystal, 1986; Butler, 1988) so that rigidity is discouraged.

The second year

If mother and child have arrived at his first birthday with confidence in each other as communicators, the way is well prepared for the next phase. As the first words start to appear it will be easier for parents to support and extend language. The ensuing years which see the transition from non-linguistic to linguistic communication will be dominated by the child's struggle to convey meaning. This will involve the negotiation of failed messages (Golinkoff, 1983). The solving of phonological problems and the achievement of early grammar are stimulated by the need to convey meaning to someone who does not have immediate, total comprehension of what you are about. The child also needs to acquire vocabulary to suit his expanding world.

Crystal (1986) and Rescorla (1984) have indicated the categories of words that young children use. The enormous amount of physical activity in which they indulge stimulates interest in action words. Their physical needs and preferences lead to rapid learning of names for different foods, clothing and parts of the body. Their individual environments will prompt the need for animal names, names of friends and relatives and names for different kinds of vehicles. Words signifying location, specificity, description and possession will emerge as soon as the child starts to combine words. Given that the child has normal abilities, good relationships and plenty of things to see and do, there is little need for advice on how to promote language. The child will dictate and the parents respond, elaborate, extend, support and puzzle out his meaning. It is only when something is lacking in the child or in the language support system that advice on how to nourish and stimulate language must be given.

Guidelines

Language guidance will try to put the mother and child in touch with each other in order that the kind of interaction and communication that take place normally can be established. Advisers will try to dissuade parents from thinking about chronological age and the arbitrary standards this dictates, and draw attention to the child's developmental level. Language cannot emerge until prelinguistic communication has taken place. The play rituals and simple auditory stimulation suitable to early infancy may be demonstrated and advocated. If these are successful, subsequent advice will make use of tactics derived from 'motherese':

● Establish a joint focus.
● Let the child determine this focus.
● Use simple, lively language to identify, describe and comment.
● Use questions and supply answers until the child is able to respond.
● Be sensitive to the child's signals both of response and of intention.
● Respond immediately to communicative signals.
● As the child becomes more adept at signalling, make the response contingent upon certain standards, e.g. if words are attempted, reward the attempt; later you may hold out until the approximation is clearer.
● Adapt your speech to the child's developing level of comprehension.
● Elaborate, extend and support the child's statement to affirm its meaning.
● Recast statements in a slightly different form in order to accelerate learning.

The important points to convey are that all situations can be used for language development and that language emerges from context. There is no need to discuss the theory of language development if mothers are happy to accept demonstrations and become successful in finding ways of their own. If mothers or caregivers wish for more information, it can be provided. Weistuch and Byers Brown (1987) report upon a programme of language facilitation in which different groups of mothers were involved. One group of mothers whose children were language delayed preferred not to explore the literature because they were upset by comparisons between their own children and children who learnt language more quickly and easily. Other groups welcomed reading material because it stimulated them to question and to discuss the procedures and to find their own solutions.

The third year

The third year is the one in which language delay may first show itself in a decisive manner and the one in which language disorder may be heralded. Rutter's guidance list starts by saying that children not using simple words by 24 months and/or not using phrases by 33 months need systematic investigation. This is in accord with the findings and opinions of a number of workers (see Chapter 2). Snyder-McClean and McClean (1987) writing about early intervention say that the diagnosis of language delay is not generally made until the child reaches the age at which at least some language production is normally expected – at least 2 years. These authors also say that the diagnosis is made on the basis of discrepancy between overall level of language development and overall level of cognitive or mental development. By contrast, language disability or language disorder are terms only applied to children who have reached a level of development characterised by the production of multi-word utterances, in other words children above the age of 3 years and who manifest very specific discrepancies within their overall linguistic perform-ance level. There is some relationship here to another of Rutter's guidelines: attention should be paid to the course of language develop-ment. Once the child has started to use words, is progress moving rapidly ahead on all fronts or is the speed of acquisition less than it should be?

The third year is the one that is probably the most significant from the prophylactic aspect since it gives us the chance to advise about delays and observe development within the framework of advice and support. How should this best be done?

Cooper, Moodley and Reynell (1978) in their well known text on *Helping Language Development* offer a developmental approach which they consider suitable for children between the ages of 2 and 4 years although it can be used for slightly older children. A major tenet is the creating of a language environment for the child. Consequently parents figure prominently and are indeed integral to the programmes. Warner, Byers Brown and McCartney (1984) give examples of how to work with the child, or the child and parent on an individual basis. Bath (1981) describes an approach to assessment and remediation carried out through the cooperation of the staff of day nurseries. Weistuch and Byers Brown (1987) offer a study showing how mothers were encouraged to assist their children's language development by modifying their own. This therapy through motherese is considered suitable as a single method or one that could be combined with other forms of therapy such as the overall developmental stimulation given in the US Early Intervention/Infant Stimulation programmes.

Early intervention programmes

Currently, educational programmes and related services are available throughout the USA through a combination of federal and state funding. A major piece of legislature was the passing of Public Law 94-142, the Education for All Handicapped Children Act. A subsequent amendment (1986) has extended provision to cover infants and toddlers as well as preschool children. Since those who work with very young children are continuously being challenged to demonstrate their effectiveness, it is heartening to read the first two items of the 1986 revision.

> P L.99-457
> Sec. 671 (a) Findings – the congress finds that there is an urgent and substantial need
> (1) to enhance the development of handicapped infants and toddlers and to minimize their potential for developmental delay,
> (2) to reduce the educational costs to our society, including our nation's schools, by minimizing the need for special education and related services after handicapped infants and toddlers reach school age.

Since the demands for accountability in the USA are extremely high, these items indicate the very real effectiveness of early intervention for children with or at risk for developmental disabilities. The programmes supported by this legislation are available for the young handicapped. In order to qualify for admission there must be demonstrable delay in at least two areas; cognitive, motor, sensory, socio-emotional and communication/language. Children with speech delay only would not qualify, nor would the programme be suitable. Indeed, some mothers refuse to enrol their children in the programmes when their main complaint is language delay because they do not want the term 'handicapped' to be attached to them. Children admitted to these programmes receive the attention of an interdisciplinary team and the emphasis is upon assisting all aspects of development. Thus the children are assessed by the whole team and developmental profiles interpretable to professionals and parents are drawn up. Parents are involved at all stages since a declared aim of the early intervention movement is to assist parents in responding to the needs of their developmentally handicapped children and to be sensitive to the changing nature of these needs (see Guralnick and Bennett (1987) for full discussion of the aims and achievements of the early intervention programmes).

Much of the philosophy and many of the procedures of the American early intervention programmes will be familiar to British workers. Working with the parents of handicapped children has been a well recognised sphere of professional activity since the early 1960s and of course, in individual circumstances, long before. Speech therapists have been very much influenced by such writers and teachers as Dorothy Jeffree and Roy McConkey. However, there is a distinctive national difference in that the American emphasis is upon intervention for all children at risk regardless of what that risk is. Thus within the same programme one might encounter children with cognitive delays, motor impairments, language/communication delays, autism and sensory impairments of hearing and vision. While each child will receive an individual assessment and programme, these will be carried out within the group structure and administered by interdisciplinary or, indeed, transdisciplinary teams.

One advantage of exposing the child to a number of highly trained professionals is that his development will be very closely observed. One would therefore expect that the language-disordered child would start to become evident. According to Rutter's guidelines, the child at risk for language disorder would be well placed within such a multidisciplinary establishment since, in addition to the language features he may display unusual or deviant motor development, socio-emotional or behavioural problems and associated medical problems. It is obviously extremely desirable for mothers that their children should receive treatment in one place and from a team of specialists each member of which is highly conversant with the methods and opinions of the others. Nevertheless objections can be made. Not all children need such a concentration of expertise and it is, of course, very expensive. In choosing a number of activities to suit all children there is very real danger of coming up with some that suit none of them. It is very difficult to keep up with the research and activities pertinent to any particular area when working all the time in a transdisciplinary capacity. Like all good endeavours, the Early Intervention Program may be saluted by those who work in other settings without the compulsion to adopt it. The UK has managed to achieve some excellent results through a combination of early therapy and special nursery placement. The NHS allows infants to receive this therapy at any age. In view of the individual variation in language development, it is very fitting that different approaches be attempted. However, in view of the similarities in their needs, it is essential that all such approaches involve the parents or caregivers.

The position paper on the role and responsibility of speech therapists in child language disability (College of Speech Therapists, 1988a) makes the following provisions:

- When language development predominantly complements an overall developmental delay, the speech therapist may monitor progress on a review basis to ensure that appropriate development continues and prevent problems arising for a child who is known to be at risk.
- When receptive and/or expressive language development is significantly delayed in relation to other skill areas, the speech therapist is more actively involved and may provide appropriate materials/programmes for parents and teachers to use with the child; progress requires to be monitored regularly by the speech therapist; periods of regular therapy may be indicated.
- When the aetiological factor is pervasive, it may conceal a language disability or prevent the development of communication; the speech therapist will monitor progress in order to form a diagnosis and decide on appropriate intervention, as for example in some cases of learning disorder or profound mental handicap.

It is important to remember that this is quoted from a position paper and not from a text on how to work with language-delayed or disordered children. Nevertheless some points may be made in relation to monitoring. It is only too easy for monitoring to become periodic assessment where the therapist carries out tests and asks questions of the parent and then provides information as to whether or not the child has progressed. To monitor is to keep a watch over. It should involve thorough discussion with the parents who may be asked to keep diaries, recordings or vocabulary lists. It involves the demonstration of ways in which language can be stimulated and suggestions as to the best times and places in which to do this. It should recommend all the normal activities through which language can be enriched at the developmental level of the child. Sometimes the parent and therapist may experiment with some material which is not immediately obvious and keep records of reactions. An interesting example of the response of a handicapped child to unusual language stimulation can be seen in Dorothy Butler's second book *Cushla and Her Books* (1987). Butler recounts the way in which a book-based compensatory programme was used for her grandchild who was developmentally handicapped. The outstanding feature of this text is in showing how something of profound importance to a family, namely reading, could be used to assist the integration and development of a child who might have been deemed unable to participate. The interest in books is central to the whole family and so uniquely useful as a language teaching method.

During the process of monitoring, the therapist may be able to find out about the interests of the family and suggest ways in which these can be shared with the child in such a way as to extend his primitive language skills. The child's response will give further clues upon which the next phase of activity may be based. This early prophylactic period is thus one in which the whole family may be prepared for long-term help and the therapist may find out what kind of help is likely to be needed. When a more thorough assessment of language skills is subsequently carried out, the parents will have been fully prepared for it and so will the child.

Some indication of the positive effects of this kind of language monitoring upon the family of the language-delayed child is given in the following account. The child in question was developmentally delayed and unresponsive with the most severe aspect of the delay being language and communication. He subsequently showed evidence of semantic–pragmatic language disorder with good powers of repetition but difficulties in comprehension and word meaning. His mother writes:

> These visits [to the language clinic] were a source of enjoyment to J. but to me they were much more. These sessions were like an infusion of energy and hope for the future. Each week we had something positive and concrete to work on at home. Life became more structured. These were times of fun and noise and great enthusiasm. I sometimes think that I benefitted even more than J. did for here I met with a positive and optimistic attitude which was just the remedy for the despondency I had experienced during the last eighteen months. These precious hours were morale boosters, and probably one of the most important factors in helping the family recover from what had seemed to be a major disaster.

At this stage of prevention, the therapist is concerned, above all, to help the family to come together and to find confidence through interaction. The discovery that a child may be handicapped is shocking and when the long-term consequences are not predictable no one knows how to behave. Prevention operates to reduce abnormal interactions that come about through anxiety and doubt. This in turn allows the normal human resourcefulness to come into being and members of the family start coming up with helpful activities. In talking about this kind of prevention, we are recognising that a comprehensive assessment of the language-delayed child's abilities and deficits may not have taken place and the measures advocated prepare everyone for this assessment. Following it, the process of tertiary prevention may be started. This will be discussed in our text following the chapter on assessment and chapters dealing more specifically with the nature of language disorders.

Older children

Work with the school-aged child is likely to be remedial rather than prophylactic except in so much as intervention at one level may reduce complications later on. It may facilitate another level of language learning. In a text devoted to written language difficulties (Snowling, 1985a), Bryant (1985) poses questions about prevention. Indeed, he asks the rather simple and basic question as to whether or not steps can be taken before the vulnerable child starts school which will allow him to pick up the skills which are necessary to avoid becoming a dyslexic. Bryant refers to the experimental studies, case histories and epidemiological surveys that have been carried out to enrich our knowledge and notes that no one has posed the question: How can we stop the problem in the first place? Bryant reviews evidence to support or negate the idea that dyslexic children form a group that is qualitatively different from other children. He comes down in favour of the continuum of reading ability with the dyslexics at the bottom end. This, he thinks is encouraging since it implies that what helps everyone will help them. 'So we just help them all.' Bryant then suggests that the best way to help them all is to improve the skill with sounds in words. He refers to the wealth of evidence that suggests that this is a skill that can be fostered and enjoyed. He suggests that we encourage our preschool children to listen to nursery rhymes and poems and then to make up their own poems. This is entirely in accord with the advice we would give to assist spoken language. Snowling, in her editorial summing up at the end of the volume, makes it clear that there are opposing views to Bryant's. Nevertheless she affirms that early intervention and training in sounds is effective even though there may still be a hard core of dyslexics not amenable to such methods.

Locke (1989), writing about the Birmingham schools programme, points out that a large number of children entering school are shown to have poor communication skills. During the primary intervention period, emphasis is placed upon the development of oral language 'Children promote their own learning through language, talking to themselves and others as they meet new experiences. Talking should be seen as a fundamental way in which children clarify their ideas and solve problems.' This activity may be seen as both prophylactic and diagnostic since it will soon throw up those children who have special communicative needs. As Beveridge and Conti-Ramsden (1987) point out, there will be differences between the degrees of skill children bring to language learning. Differences in children's memory, verbal reasoning abilities, inferential abilities and verbal playfulness are all mentioned as being important. The skilled teacher can do much to encourage all these attributes and thus promote interest and confidence in language learning and in language use.

Chapter 4
The Nature of Language Disorders: How may they be described?

Summary

This chapter begins with a general outline of principles of information processing. It then continues by discussing the possible application of such a model to neurobiological, cognitive and linguistic aspects of language. Ways in which impairment or inefficiency of processing may contribute to developmental language disorders are considered.

It is essential if we are to come to terms with the entire range of language disorders that we should be able to see them in relation to a theoretical model which may offer cohesion and indicate relationships. This chapter will therefore discuss the neurobiological, psycholinguistic and linguistic aspects of language disorder within the context of language processing.

Because each is described separately, it would be misleading to deduce that they are discrete. Rather, they represent different facets of the same coin, namely language. There are obvious overlaps and interactions between them. Psycholinguistic aspects, for example, form a bridge between neuropsychology and linguistics, and cognitive aspects are linked both to physiology and psychology. The emphasis on the eclectic nature of these models is important for it is noticeable that much of the literature takes an exclusive stance often in favour of one model and, depending on the viewpoint of the writer, with accompanying criticism of others. Before a more detailed consideration of these models some preliminary description of the principles of information processing may be beneficial as this provides a framework in which to consider the special place of language.

Essentially information processing as has been described in Chapter 1 can be reduced to a very simple level in which there are three main components:

1. A receiver.

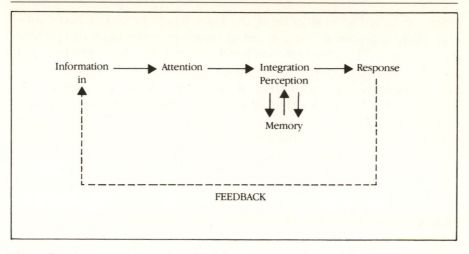

Figure 4.1 Schematic representation of an information processing model.

2. A control system
3. An effector.

A simple model of this type has immediate application to the case of Stephen described in the first chapter. The human being as the processor is seen to play an active part, that is to say, he is not a passive recipient of incoming information. Stelmach (1982) postulates some important assumptions which underlie information processing.

First is the fact that there are many stages between the reception of the incoming stimulus and the subsequent response. In fact, the nature of the response may be of minor significance in the processing chain, for it will have been predetermined by the previous stages, although a number of options will have been available.

Secondly, the sequence of events is invariable, for each stage can only operate on information received from the previous stimulus. The notion of a control system operating in the absence of a receiver is ludicrous. The ringing of a telephone bell for example, has first to be detected and recognised before being answered, in that order.

Thirdly, each stage effects change in the information it receives; this is an event which takes time.

Finally, once processing at a particular stage is complete, the information is made available to the next stage.

A simple model of information processing is given in Figure 4.1.

Attention

As human beings we are constantly bombarded with incoming information from the environment – sights, sounds, smells, movement etc. – were we to attempt to attend to all of these, the result would be one of utter confusion. There is a limit to the amount of information the brain can process at any one time. G. Miller (1967) in his eloquent essay, 'The magical number of 7 plus or minus 2' refers to the information bottleneck which can only be overcome by the organisation of incoming material into manageable sequential chunks or units. This of course is closely related to memory.

Moray (1972) describes a theory of capacity attention which also suggests an overall limit to the amount of information to which the system can attend, regardless of the number of channels involved. This means that up to a capacity point, multimodal attention is possible, but once past that point, there will be decrement in processing ability. This theory is of interest when one considers the low threshold of multimodal attention in some language-disordered children.

Moray's views are in conflict with another major theory of attention, that proposed by Broadbent in 1958. In order to avoid the problem of an overloaded system he suggested that the only way in which information can be handled is sequentially. Earlier stages of detection and recognition, he maintained, can take place without attention so that, peripherally, multichannels can carry information in parallel. In order to process two simultaneous messages, one is transferred to the short-term memory store. The longer it is held there, the greater is its degradation. Obviously there is a strong element of selectivity in such an operation. This will relate to the strength of the stimulus and also to the subject's familiarity with it.

Whichever model is favoured, it is accepted that attention plays a crucial part in language acquisition.

Perception

Incoming information is held briefly in memory storage [approximately 200–300 ms according to Haber and Standing (1969) quoted by Stelmach (1972)], before it is perceived. Hebb (1972) emphasises the point that perception is more than complex sensation. Presumably it is the activity of mediating processes which result from sensory input. Luria (1973) describes it as the encoding and synthesis of incoming information which is then compared with previous experience. This definition also implies a close association with memory. It may be speculated that this is a point of extreme vulnerability for the developing child. Instances of shaky motor coordination come to mind as, for example, children's early attempts at hopping, climbing stairs, throwing and catching. While the results are manifest in motor response, the mismatch arises from an as yet incomplete synthesis of visual, tactile and proprioceptive input.

Memory

Stelmach (1982) describes three functions associated with memory: *encoding, storage* and *retrieval*. Encoding is the stage whereby percepts undergo transformation for storage. This information is then stored over a period of time. At one time memory was described as a two-part process: short term and long term. Current views, however, favour the notion of it being on a continuum which differs qualitatively. Partly corresponding to short-term memory, though not exclusively so, is episodic or working memory. This has been likened to an internal diary which records day-to-day factual events many of which do not need to be retained. Most auditory memory tasks are designed to test this. Conceptual or semantic memory is the internal dictionary. This, as the name suggests, stores concepts and meaning. Episodic memory is vulnerable to decay, but it can, through strategies of rehearsal and reinforcement, be transferred to the greater permanence of conceptual memory. It is generally agreed that there are four types of code involved in memory storage: *iconic*, *symbolic*, *verbal* and *motor*. In relation to language, it will be seen that all these codes have an important role and their strengths will be discussed further on p.100.

Retrieval includes the accessing and extrapolation of information from memory. Bruner (1964) describes it as being the most important stage of the language process. Luria (1973) states that retrieval is active and complex in nature. In recalling information, the individual is required to select, from the storage codes, that which is most appropriate for the task in hand. Increasing attention has in recent years been focused on *forgetting*. Whereas it was formerly thought that memory traces simply faded with the passage of time, it has been shown that interference has a deleterious effect on retention. Stelmach, Kelso and Wallace (1975) carried out a study in which subjects were taught a new movement. During the period of rehearsal immediately following, half the sample was assigned a distracting task (counting). There was poorer retention of the movement in these subjects than in the controls. There is an obvious correspondence here with the difficulties which highly distractable children experience in retaining information.

Response

This entails, first, appropriate selection from memory and, secondly, the planning and programming of whichever type of response best fits the event; this may be motor or verbal. In the selection process, the individual must take into account contextual factors, as, for example, the environment, to ensure efficacy. Information about such efficacy is conveyed through two main processes: *feedback* and *feedforward*.

Feedback

There are two major divisions which operate. These are open and closed loop. In the former, the previous processes preset the conditions and no peripheral influence is exerted until the act is completed. Closed loop is exemplified in the model described by Fairbanks in 1954 which relates

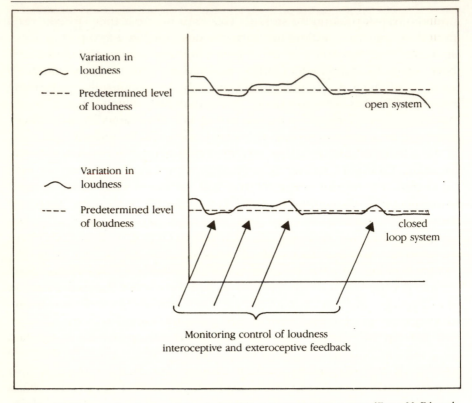

Variation in loudness

- - - - Predetermined level of loudness

open system

Variation in loudness

- - - - Predetermined level of loudness

closed loop system

Monitoring control of loudness
interoceptive and exteroceptive feedback

Figure 4.2 Diagram showing opened and closed loop programming system. (From M. Edwards (1984) *Disorders of Articulation,* Vienna, Springer-Verlag.)

specifically to speech, but which is an adaptation of a servo-system model. This includes an ongoing monitoring facility as sensory information is fed into the system from the motor activity which is generated. Figure 4.2 shows a schematic representation of the two types of feedback.

Feedforward

This has an anticipatory function. As motor programmes are built up during early development, there is as a consequence some degree of preplanning of the perceptual system. Thus comparison can be made at each stage between incoming information and the established pattern so that control is exercised on the response before it becomes overt. Feedforward may therefore be described as an internal monitoring system which has a capability of detecting errors prior to output.

Kelso (1982) states that both feedback and feedforward are essential for skilled performance. Their function is interactive. He quotes as illustration an example cited by Arbib (1972). When we are walking on familiar ground or descending a known staircase, there is no necessity to 'test' the ground ahead; the feedforward process operates on the basis of past familiarity and experience of the action. On unfamiliar ground, however, there is a need to explore so that information regarding changes of surface, possible obstacles etc. can be fed back and the necessary adjustments made. This description represents a very simplified model of information processing, but nevertheless it is one which it is possible to apply to some aspects of language processing. Criticisms of the model include a charge of reductionism and to some extent, considering the complexity of language, this may be true. It is also said that it pays too little heed to the importance of cognitive aspects and also to the impingement of the environment on the individual. Sufficient allowance is also not made for the effects of learning.

There is, however, the possibility of including cognitive strategies within such a model which reduces the criticism of automaticity. In relation to the development of memory, for example, Brown (1975) has shown that conscious cognitive strategies will effect progress. Hubbell (1981) describes human information processing as 'a dynamic multiply determined adaptable system response to both outside stimuli and to its own functions' (p.39).

Neurobiological aspects of language processing

Language represents a synthesis of psychological, linguistic and physiological behaviours (Edwards, 1984). In this section we consider the neurophysiological system which underlies language.

Language is received through two principal sensory channels: *auditory* and *visual*. Spoken language relies mainly on the former although concomitant information is relayed along visual channels through gesture, facial expression etc. For written language to be understood, an intact visual sensory channel is necessary, although this again may be enhanced through the medium of accompanying auditory stimuli. To a lesser extent (other than in the case of visually impaired children), touch plays a secondary role. The importance of *proprioceptive channels* is a subject of ongoing debate. Liberman and his colleagues published a classic paper in 1967 in which they claimed that proprioceptive feedback was an essential component of comprehension, but conflicting evidence is provided by instances of anarthric children with well developed comprehension (Christopher Nolan is one outstanding example). It is most likely that proprioceptive channels act mainly to ensure maintenance of speech, while auditory pathways play a very important part in language acquisition. The respective roles of the two modes of input is well illustrated in the case of remedial programmes for people with acquired hearing loss. Segmental aspects of speech can be maintained to some extent through tactile and proprioceptive input, but non-segmental (prosodic) elements pose difficulties and reliance then has to be placed on visual models as in the use of instrumentation such as Visispeech.

Reception of information

The central nervous system structures governing the reception of incoming information may be divided into primary and secondary cortical regions. Taking the auditory system as a starting point, afferent impulses from the organ of Corti in the inner ear travel via the reticular system to the primary auditory cortex. Within the reticular system which is also concerned with attention, preliminary selection and inhibition of input takes place. Mysack (1976) describes this lower order receptor system as having three functions: the orienting of the head to the source of the signal, stimulating arousal mechanisms and generating efferent impulses to regulate the responsiveness of the auditory system at any level. This last function is effected through descending nerve fibres which provide

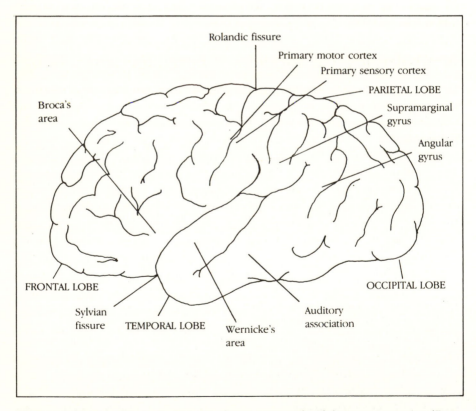

Figure 4.3 Diagram of brain showing site of areas concerned with language processing. (From M. Edwards (1984) *Disorders of Articulation,* Vienna, Springer-Verlag.)

feedback so that adjustments can be made to the incoming stimuli at points along the tract in the many relay stations (nuclei).

All ascending fibres of the eighth cranial nerve (cochlear division) pass through the thalamus via the medial geniculate body and it is thought that further refinement of the signal takes place at this level. Within the cerebral cortex, Luria (1970) describes three zones which are essential to auditory perception. The first is the *primary projection area* which lies deep in the temporal lobe within Heschl's gyrus. This part is said to contain cells which are specifically adapted to respond to certain frequencies of sound. This has led some workers to speculate that early feature discrimination may take place here. Geschwind and Levitsky (1968) have noted that this particular zone is larger in the left (dominant) side than in the right.

The second cortical unit is the *association temporal cortex* which lies in the superior posterior temporal region (the classic Wernicke's area). Its function is concerned with the refinement, recognition and synthesis of signals which have already received primary analysis in the projection cortex. It is likely that at this point, phonological coding takes place including features of sequence and timing. The listener is thus enabled to recognise, for example, subtle allophonic variations. From this area a pathway runs in the arcuate fasciculus forward to Broca's area which is the association cortex lying anterior to the motor strip concerned with movement for speech. The association temporal cortex has an important role in relation to episodic memory storage. This it shares with the hippocampus, but it is thought that long-term (semantic) memory is stored throughout the brain.

Integration

The function of the third unit is that of integration of perceptions from the different modalities. Anatomically this lies at the junction of the auditory, visual and somaesthetic association cortices. This has been called 'the association area of association areas' – it is the angular gyrus, occurs only in humans and is one of the later parts of the brain to become myelinated. Figure 4.3 shows the anatomical location of these areas.

Geschwind states that myelination may not take place much before the age of 5 years. Since intermodal coding is considered to be essential for language development this supports Lenneberg's (1967) description of language development as a gradual progressive unfolding in which morphological and physiological events play a highly influential part. Luria calls this region the *tertiary zone*.

Innervation is bilateral for hearing, but experimental evidence derived from many studies usually involving dichotic listening tasks indicates that the dominant hemisphere is the main processor of linguistic input, although, to a lesser extent, the non-dominant hemisphere does partici-pate. There is a possibility that a change in this pattern occurs where damage is sustained in infancy, but there is a fair amount of variation expressed in views about the extent to which the assumption of the language role is taken over by the non-dominant hemisphere (see, for example, Woods and Carey, 1979).

So far in this discussion of the neurophysiology of language we have paralleled the information processing model in relation to input, attention, integration and storage. We now need to consider response, that is to say, how is language actually produced? Between perception and ideation and between ideation – the germ of an idea of what we want to say (according to Lashley, 1951) – and the onset of speech there are gaps which at the present time remain unbridged. Obviously, before any programming of language can take place, there must be an intention to speak. This may well be generated as a result of external factors, but it can equally well be triggered by emotion (Mountcastle, 1980).

Production

Planning of an utterance entails the preparation of schemata which best fit the requirements of the linguistic programme. Such schemata are built up during language development through the integration of incoming sensory information. They correspond to the integrated percepts which have been described above.

At one time it was thought that each movement (in this context, concerned with speech) was stored as an individual unit in the cerebral cortex, so that by exciting specific pyramidal cells, a particular movement would ensue. The cerebral cortex was seen as a master controller. Such an ingenuous theory is patently unacceptable in the light of current knowledge when one considers the complexity and variation which attends the production of even a single sound especially if one takes into account allophonic features. The idea that the brain, even acknowledging its vast neuronal structure, could store such an amount of information, is beyond imagination. Wickelgren (1969), for example, proposed a theory which included the storage of context-sensitive allophones, each of which would slot into only one phonetic environment. Allowing for variations this would necessitate storage of over 100 000 separate items – again an untenable idea.

Problems relating to storage led the psychologist Hebb in 1949 to propose a theory of *motor equivalence*. During the learning of an activity, integrated percepts from auditory, visual and proprioceptive channels are built up to form internalised patterns of that activity. This is not a detailed plan, but an overall schema which is directed towards the target. There is therefore allowance for possible variation in the circumstances in which the target is reached. A good example is that where a person can speak intelligibly while a pipe is clutched between the teeth. To achieve this there must be a series of adaptive movements of tongue and lips to allow for the relative immobility of the jaws. A more striking example is the degree of intelligibility achieved by patients following partial glossectomies and this also is the result of compensatory movements designed to meet a target.

These internalised patterns are stored in semantic memory to be utilised to meet the needs of the linguistic programme.

The fundamental goals are defined at cortical level, but the coordinative action necessary for speech production is the outcome of multilevel activity within the central nervous system. Important points of control would be at cerebellar, subcortical and brain stem levels. This hierarchy represents a consensus rather than a central executive mode of control. The basis of this model of speech production derives first from the theory of motor equivalence proposed by Hebb and extensively developed by MacNeilage (1970) and then from the work of the Russian physiologist Bernstein, who in 1967 described movement as being divided into 'functional units whose precise combination represents coordinate action' (p.91).

Subcortical systems

Some of the thalamic nuclei act as coordinators of the three cortical areas referred to above (Penfield and Roberts, 1959). They are also concerned with the ordering and motivational aspects of speech (Purpura and Yahr, 1966) through their connections with the motor cortex. A regulatory influence on movement is exercised by the basal ganglia which act as an interconnecting circuit between the cerebral cortex and the thalamus. Impairment of function may give rise to disfluencies of speech production.

The cerebellar system

The cerebellum functions as a modifier and refiner of the descending motor schemata. This is achieved through the preponderance of input fibres; the ratio of input to output is said to be about 40:1. The sensory information contained serves to monitor the relatively unrefined motor commands which issue from the cerebral cortex. The controlling effect of this function becomes apparent when one considers the superfluity of movement which is a feature of cerebellar disease. The initiation and termination of speech control over pause and stress are all thought to lie within its domain. Eccles (1973) considers it to be the seat of all complicated movement and that 'throughout life we are engaged in an incessant teaching programme for the cerebellum' (p.123).

Transmission

Transmission of impulses along nervous pathways is an electrochemical process which entails a shift between negative and positive charges. In unmyelinated fibres the flow of current is smooth and relatively slow, but where myelination has occurred, this acts as an insulator and transmission is much faster. In order to prevent the inhibition of flow, the myelin sheath is interrupted at regular intervals (the nodes of Ranvier) to allow for the chemical change of ionisation.

Myelination allows for the more rapid conduct of current. Most of the cranial nerves which serve the vocal tract are myelinated, but this is far from complete at birth. There is a direct relationship between language acquisition and myelination of the higher centres of the central nervous system. Netsell (1986) suggests that the most sensitive period for acquisition of motor control of speech appears to be between 3;0 and 12;0 months and this is also a period of rapid myelination of the nerve tracts. Delays during this time, he considers, may have serious implications for the normal development of coordination of movement within the vocal tract. It is during this stage that the fundamental schemata for speech patterns begin to be laid down.

Neurotransmitters exert considerable influence on interneural connections. This is either facilitatory or inhibitory. One of the most frequently cited effects is the resulting dysarthria occurring when dopaminergic cells are destroyed. Coyle (1983), quoted by Netsell, stated that if autistic children do develop language, this takes place at about 4–5 years of age and this is at a time when serotonin, a powerful vasoconstrictor, increases markedly in the brain. Netsell observes that this is also a time when children acquire finer control over motor speech.

In relation to development of the brain, Dobbing (1972) emphasises three major factors. The first is its comparatively large size in relation to the body at birth, the second is the early growth spurt and the third is the achievement of mature size at an early stage compared with the rest of the body. The rapid growth extends from the last 10 weeks of fetal life to about 2 years of age. By the last 13 weeks, the adult number of neurones is present. The subsequent growth spurt, therefore, is concerned with the building up of interneuronal connections, with the increase of oligodendrial cells which manufacture myelin sheaths and with the synthesis of the constituents of myelin. Possible deleterious consequences of interruption of the growth spurt have been discussed in Chapter 2.

Cognitive processing of language

The relationship between cognition and language is not at all clear cut. In fact, Campbell (1979) prefaces a chapter on this subject by describing it as 'a very dark forest indeed. It is not so much a question of not being able to see the wood for the trees: one cannot even see the trees!' (p. 419).

Rice (1983) writing a response to a paper on cognition/language relationship states:

> Questions concerning the relationship of cognition and language are not susceptible of empirical resolution, because definitions in the literature of 'language' and 'cognition' are too fluid and imprecise.

The place of cognition as an underpinning of language has, as one of its chief proponents, the work of Piaget and that of his many followers. We will return to consider this further on in this chapter.

The antithesis of this view is that expressed by Skinner in 1957. It must be stated, however, that some of the reproach which attended the publication of this work was based on a misunderstanding of some of the claims made by the author. It is true that in terms of the theory of operant conditioning, he saw language learning as the result of shaping and reinforcement, but he did not extend this to the learning of every utterance. Basic units could be combined to form new utterances. Nevertheless, any element of creativity is palpably lacking in this theory.

Perception and recognition

Pursuing the information processing model previously described, we need to consider features which influence the perception of spoken input, the changes which take place on its reception and possible storage strategies. Cognitive strategies also need to be developed to deal effectively with incoming information. Hubbell (1981) defines this term as representing 'a continuum from very automatic activity that may occur almost without awareness . . . . . . to very conscious purposive activity such as that employed in various types of problem solving' (p. 37). These strategies may differ in individuals, for they are learned and may therefore be acquired in different circumstances both within the child and through the environment.

Memory plays an intrinsic part in the development of cognition and children have to develop critical selection and means of retention of relevant stimuli from the environment. This development is largely involuntary, but experimental work has shown it to be more effective where the input is meaningful. Language acts as a powerful reinforcer for retention and in turn it would be difficult to consider language without memory. Children with severe learning difficulties may be taught specific strategies for remembering, but they are limited by their inability to apply these, other than to a particular learned situation. Craig and Tulving (1975) examined processes by which retention of memory might take place. They provided a number of stimulus words and asked the subjects to process each one according to a different dimension. In the case of written words they were required to visualise the physical characteristics of size, length etc; another type of processing involved the phonological properties of the word and a third focused on meaning. They found there was a significant relationship between the type of processing and the retention of words. Those that were best retained were associated with meaning. The children were required to reflect on the meaning and to relate this to semantic memory. This effect was consistent throughout a series of 10 studies.

The sensory stimulus itself may not be sufficient to lead to recognition. It is dependent on context, previous experience and expectation. Pragmatic factors also play an important role. As language develops, these elements all need to be acquired, for the young child starts with a limitation of knowledge of the world including his native language. St Augustine in *Confessions Book 1* provides a vivid account of his growing awareness as a young child of the importance of language:

> . . . . . . I noticed that people would name some object and then turn towards whatever it was they had named. I watched them and understood that the sound they made when they wanted to indicate that particular thing was the name which they gave to it . . . .   *Confessions Book 1*

In the case of language-disordered children such knowledge will be even more poorly defined. As well as being adjuncts to recognition, context, experience and prediction also act to speed up processing.

Coltheart (1987) in a discussion of language processing in adults, describes a model which has affinities with Morton's (1978) work on logogens and which has been developed by Marslen-Wilson and Tyler (1980). This is known as the cohort model.

At the input level, there is an auditory word recognition system (there are also comparable visual and picture written systems, but these do not concern us here). This is connected to a semantic–cognitive system which acts as a storage resource. This in turn is connected to a production system. The schematic representation of this model as presented by Coltheart is shown in Figure 4.4.

The word recognition system includes a series of word detectors which can be potentially equally activated. When a spoken stimulus occurs an immediate process of analysis starts. Suppose the stimulus is the word 'play'. As soon as the phoneme /p/ is detected all the words *not* beginning with this will be inactivated; similarly when the next element of the cluster /l/ is recognised, further elimination will take place leaving only those likely candidates which have /pl/ in initial position. This process of analysis continues until the word is complete or recognised. Obviously in many cases it will not be necessary to go through the entire range of detectors for recognition to take place; in such instances context and experience act as facilitators. Highly predictable utterances such as 'Happy Christmas' will be recognised very early on. The model is extended to include analysis of discourse and, to accommodate this, concurrent syntactic and semantic analysis are thought to take place. There is some doubt about the actual boundaries involved. It is suggested that these may be clausal. It is also not clear whether there is a preliminary phonological analysis followed by a semantic/syntactic sweep. There is, however, a strongly defined interactive component between the levels.

This model favours a top-down processing strategy in that it is influenced by previous knowledge and prediction.

Bottom-up processing relies on recognition of sound patterns through acoustic cues received.

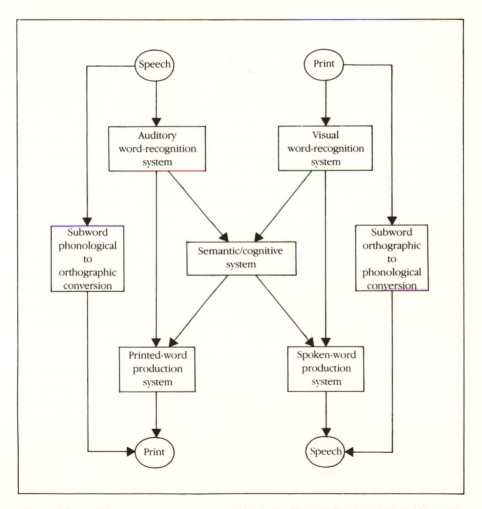

Figure 4.4 An information processing model of language. (From M. Harris and M. Coltheart, Eds (1987) *Language Processing in Children and Adults*, London, Routledge, Keegan & Paul.)

Both methods interact. This can be illustrated by examples of semantic errors. For instance, one student referred consistently in a written paper to a 'Raw Shark' (Rorscharch) test. She had analysed the acoustic sequence correctly (bottom-up), but because this word had not previously existed in her lexicon, she equated with two which did, although with minimal semantic accuracy.

Development of cognitive systems

The model described above refers principally to conditions where language has already been acquired. We now need to consider some of the factors underlying its acquisition.

In the first instance, development of attention is necessary. Theories of attention have been discussed in the first section of this chapter. Kagan (1971) proposed three stages: the first is that of total attention which is, however, fleeting and which decreases rapidly as the object is removed and interest fades. This would coincide with pre-object permanence in Piagetian terms. The second stage is that which he terms 'discrepancy'; this is when some discordant feature is introduced into the situation and this serves to sharpen attention. The third stage is that of density of stimuli. Here the individual is able to integrate different stimuli to produce novel experiences.

Semantic memory serves as the storage system; this corresponds to the semantic cognitive system referred to above. Wickelgren (1979) defines semantic memory as the means whereby incoming information from whatever modality, is coded in abstract. This is more or less similar to the traditional notion of long-term memory. The information which is stored, as well as verbal codes, includes that which relates to vision, space and movement. His model is hierarchical and proposes, in rising order of complexity, coding of concepts, propositions and schemata. There is no one-to-one correspondence with specific linguistic units, though semantic memory does appear to include the coding of linguistic information (L. Miller, 1984).

Piagetian theorists claim that concepts develop initially independent of language, i.e. they are the outcome of sensorimotor activity. Conceptual knowledge without appropriate linkage with linguistic knowledge is observed in children with predominantly expressive-type language disorders. They may be able to demonstrate that they 'know' an object and that they can differentiate it from other similar objects without being able to signal this knowledge linguistically. Take, for example, a shoe. The child can identify it by form and function. He may be able to differentiate between one shoe and more than one shoe, and from other shoes, all in the absence of knowledge of the appropriate word. The converse of this condition is when a child can use words without having developed corresponding concepts. Obviously, conceptual knowledge at this very basic level will be severely limiting. Examples of this state are seen in some of the case illustrations in Chapter 5.

At a more complex level of coding, propositional structures are thought to store information about phrases, clauses and sentences, while schemata are thought to be concerned with the encoding of discourse size pieces of spoken and written text. L. Miller (1984) attempts an analysis of children's language within the framework of the semantic memory model, but as she herself observes, this is a highly speculative endeavour. Indeed many of the models of memory discussed in the literature are based on hypotheses which are as yet unproven. One of the main obstacles is the difficulty of assessing semantic memory. Most of the tests in use apply only to episodic memory. P. Piaget views language development as an outcome of cognitive development. Early language and development of representational thought are concurrent but not interdependent (Sinclair de Zwart, 1969). There is thus a firm focus on the sensorimotor period and, in particular, on the motor component of this as a prerequisite for the development of language. In the first stage, language takes the form of illocutionary vocalisations, i.e. they accompany a motor activity. As shown earlier in this chapter, the assumption that the influence of motor activity is all pervasive has been questioned by the evidence of severely physically handicapped children developing normal levels of comprehension (Lenneberg, 1967). Piagetians would argue that a minimal amount of motor activity as, for example, eye movement would constitute sufficient experience. This does, however, appear to stretch the theory to the utmost limits. Language development is therefore regarded as one aspect of the complex of processes taking place, sharing common roots with symbolic play. Dean and Howell (1966) have combined Piagetian and metalinguistic theory as a basis for therapeutic intervention in disorders of phonology. Chapter 6 makes reference to Van Kleek's 1981 review of metalinguistic development within a Piagetian model. For Bruner, the development of language is a much more socially orientated and interactive process. Early vocalisations lead to the building of concepts and as vocabulary increases so the child finds a verbal outlet for their expression (Bruner, 1975).

Cromer (1978) suggests that language has a hierarchical structure of organisation. It is not based on a series of associative links, but each part acts in relation to the structure as a whole. This idea has certain commonalities with the Wickelgren model of semantic memory described above. Some types of language disorder can be construed as the outcome of failure of hierarchical organisation, particularly so when surface structures as, for example, relative clauses, occur. In such instances, the language-disordered child may be unable to process them and will tend to reduce them to simple elements.

The sentence: 'The horse the girl rides is fat' may become:
> 'The girl rides a horse'
> 'The girl is fat'

In such instances, careful examination is necessary to determine the point of breakdown, i.e. whether such a structure is too complex for adequate storage or whether, alternatively, the problem lies in accessing it and the constraint lies more in relation to difficulty of planning production. Had the interpretation been:

> 'The girl rides a horse'
> 'The horse is fat'

the latter explanation would have been favoured.

Retrieval

Children have to learn strategies to develop a system of retrieval from semantic memory. One such stratagem is the categorisation of incoming information into a superordinate structure so that 'dog, cat, horse etc.' would be coded under the superordinate 'animal'.

At first these categories will relate mainly to concrete objects, but with maturity, more abstract categories will be learned. In relation to association tasks too, there is evidence of maturational change. Very young children (up to around 7 years) respond to a stimulus word with one from a different syntactic category, e.g. biscuit→eat. As language develops, the response becomes paradigmatic, i.e. it is drawn from the same syntactic category: biscuit–cake–pastry (Brown and Berko, 1960). There is some evidence that language-disordered children have difficulty in making this shift and it is speculated that this may be the result of problems of reorganisation in the semantic domain.

Linguistic model of processing

It will be apparent from the foregoing discussion of aspects of human language processing that this is a field which is rife with speculation. Since the mid-1960s there has been a surge of experimental work directed towards an attempt to gain a clearer understanding of its nature. Unfortunately, the published studies have, to some extent because of conflicting findings, only served to emphasise the labyrinthine state which pertains at the present time.

It is, however, generally accepted that any investigation of language behaviour requires a framework in which to place descriptive data. This cannot occur in a vacuum and the case is even stronger when the language under investigation is aberrant. In the absence of such a model, the ultimate aim of achieving some coherence in devising a taxonomy is likely to be jeopardised.

The last section of this chapter offers a very broad model of linguistic programming. Detailed consideration is purposely omitted for the reasons given above. The intention is to provide a model sufficiently general to accommodate the factors which we know from clinical experience and from empirical work to be characteristic of developmental language disorders. The framework is an amalgam of that proposed by Laver in 1977 and Garrett in 1980. The decision to concentrate on a description of the processes which may underlie language production has been taken, because the previous sections have tended to concentrate on input and

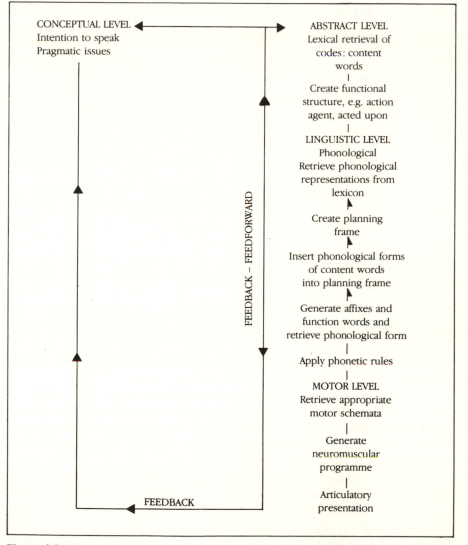

Figure 4.5 Model of language production. (Adapted from Garrett (1980) and Laver (1977) with kind permission.)

storage and also it is contended that inferences may be drawn regarding this aspect from the data on output. A schematic representation of the model is given in Figure 4.5.

At the conceptual level, the speaker gains an idea of the message which is to be conveyed. It is possible that, at this stage of planning, provision is also included for pragmatic aspects. If the utterance is part of an ongoing dialogue, feedback will have been forthcoming on listener reaction so that the response or new message will take cognisance of this.

Still at abstract level the next process is the retrieval of codes from the lexicon. These represent the content words in which the message is to be framed. Additionally, a structure for the message is created. Cognitive neuropsychology favours the terms 'argument' and 'predicate'. These are terms used in semantic theory and refer to the relationship inherent in the conceptualisation of the message. Another way of expressing this is to use the terms 'agent', 'acted upon' and 'instrument' (Coltheart, 1987).

John gave	the ball to	Mary
Agent	Instrument	Acted upon

This is not at this stage a syntactic representation for, as yet, planning has not extended to decisions regarding the syntactic form the message will take, e.g. whether passive or active.

Retrieval from semantic memory is vulnerable in that the appropriate conceptual code may be inaccessible or, because of impairment in perceptual processing, storage may not have been possible. Failure at this stage will result in severe forms of language disorder (auditory agnosia).

Linguistic processing begins with the retrieval of phonological forms of the content words. A planning frame is then created into which these are inserted. As the message now assumes a syntactic form certain function words and affixes need to be generated and then assimilated into the frame in correct sequence. This brings the processing operation to the positional level (Garrett, 1980) where it is held in its full phonological form in readiness for the application of the phonetic rules as a prelude to motor planning.

Before discussing the next stage of motor planning it may be fruitful to consider further this linguistic level with a view to the possible relation between this stage and certain types of language disorder. The complexity of the processing, and the speed at which it is carried out, obviously make for vulnerability to breakdown or impairment.

There are two further issues which merit attention. The first relates to the unit of storage in the lexicon and on this point there is little evidence of unanimity. Word, syllable and phoneme have all been cited. The model described above appears to infer storage at word level and this is supported by Shattuck-Huffnagel (1979) with the proviso already emphasised here that this is in abstract form. If words were stored in complete phonological form corresponding to surface structure, the phenomenon of slips of the tongue which occurs frequently in normal speech production, would be difficult to explain. In favour of storage at syllable level are Fromkin (1968) and Kozhevnikov and Chistovich (1965) while Liberman *et al.* (1964) opt for the phoneme as the smallest invariant unit.

The second issue is concerned with the length of speech which is preplanned at any one time. Halliday (1963) considers this to be the *tone unit.* This is a stretch of speech lasting over seven or eight syllables with a nuclear stress falling towards the end usually on a content word. This is signalled by a change in pitch direction. The tone unit acts as an 'envelope' to carry the non-segmental information about the message, i.e. rhythm, intonation and stress. It is likely that these prosodic features are encoded fairly early on in the programme since they both underlie and influence the syntactic form that the utterance will take. It is important to differentiate between prosodic disorder at this level which is *linguistic* in origin and that which arises further downstream at the neuromuscular stage which is *phonetic* in origin. Were this fact more readily recognised, there might be less controversy surrounding the nature of verbal dyspraxia. If the possibility of multifactorial levels of impairment is accepted then the idea of it being both linguistic and motor or either is perfectly compatible with observed data.

The part played by pausing in normal language production casts an interesting light on underlying processing. It is known that spoken language is well interspersed with pauses, hesitations, false starts and repetitions in even the most fluent of speakers. These are not equally spaced, but tend to occur in alternating bursts of non-fluency followed by a fluent stretch. It is thought that during the non-fluent phase there is active preplanning leading to the fluent phase. This type of pausing, of course, differs qualitatively and quantitatively from disorders of fluency arising from neurological conditions. Non-fluency is a well recognised feature of language development and it is interesting to conjecture that this condition which has in the past been attributed to vocabulary deficit may in fact reflect the child's development of language processing.

Impaired ability to retrieve content words from the lexicon will manifest itself as a word-finding difficulty. Whilst there may be adequacy of function words, indeed a superfluity at times, the circumlocutions, hesitations and repetitions can lead to almost unintelligible speech. This is a short example from a boy aged 6;6 years:

> The teacher – she had this kind kind of thing – (a pencil) and she do do p . . . drawed it.

On the other hand some children have a good range of content words but are unable to produce the appropriate syntactic framework, so that speech sounds telegraphic with a paucity of function words.

The relationship between syntax and phonological representation is critical and each one influences the other, as for example, where phonological deficits result in morphological changes.

We have described the conceptual level where the intention to speak and the pragmatic aspects are considered. It is perfectly possible to by-pass this stage of processing and still produce syntactically and phonologi-cally acceptable utterances, but the word 'utterance' is used advisedly, for there is little communicative intent apparent. These conditions will be discussed more fully in Chapter 5.

Linguistic processing is of course dependent on intact neurological function and on the development of the cognitive system. Much of the underlying neurolinguistic planning takes place at cortical level, probably partly in the association cortex, Broca's area, although current ideas do not favour the supremacy of any one region of the brain assuming complete responsibility for a specific aspect of language. It is therefore likely that other areas of the cerebral hemispheres, e.g. the supplementary motor cortex, also contribute to language processing.

Concept formation as we have seen is closely interrelated with cognitive development and where there is inadequacy in the latter this will be reflected in the former. Children with severe learning difficulties provide obvious examples of such difficulties and in such cases the language deficit may be regarded as the direct outcome of the cognitive impairment.

The *motor level* of processing begins with the retrieval of appropriate motor schemata which best fit the message. This too is an abstract process in so far as precise movements are not at this stage prescribed by higher cortical centres. Initiation probably occurs in the precentral motor strip once the linguistic components have been determined, but thereafter the planning relies on influences throughout the central nervous system. Motor schemata, as we have seen in the previous description of neurological function, are concerned with the general pattern of move-ment necessary to achieve the target. This activity is also under the control of feedback (external and internal) and of feedforward processes so that ongoing adjustments can be made at this covert level.

Impairment in neuromuscular programming may well give rise to dyspraxic-type disorders as well as to those associated with the cerebral palsies. These must be differentiated from lower motor neurone disorders where resulting impairment of the vocal tract prevents adequate produc-tion of speech. Such conditions are analogous with structural conditions such as orofacial deformities. At the same time it is important to remember that any of these conditions can co-occur with impairment at other levels in the processing chain.

The motor schemata lead to the planning of the neuromuscular programme which specifies the precise configuration of muscular activity within the entire vocal tract (including respiratory forces) deemed necessary to deliver the message which at this point becomes overt. External feedback through the sensory channels then occurs and this in turn contributes to revision and/or to the generation of a new message.

This very general description of an information processing approach to language may at times have given the impression that it occurs in a semi-vacuum unaffected by outside influences. This is erroneous for one of the main functions of language is to communicate and, in order for this to be effective, the individual has to be aware of interactive and pragmatic aspects. Similarly he has to learn to reflect on the properties of language in order to use it effectively; in other words he must develop an awareness of language.

The position of pragmatic aspects of language in relation to a processing model is problematic. There are those who regard it as underlying all communicative activity, and as the precursor of all forms of spoken language, for it provides the context in which this can take place; in other words it makes language meaningful. Certainly the truth of this is apparent when one considers the nature of semantic–pragmatic disorders. Prutting and Kirchner (1983) argue persuasively for such a view as against that which was prevalent in the late 1960s where syntax reigned supreme. In contrast to the functionalists there are those who see pragmatics as a separate level of language in parallel with phonology, syntax and semantics. Lund and Duchan (1983) regard a combination of these two views as providing the most fruitful interface between a strictly linguistic and a functional approach. Such aspects have important implications for remediation, and ways in which they can be utilised will be considered in Chapter 7.

Chapter 5
The Differentiation of Clinical Subtypes

Summary

This chapter reviews a number of studies which have contributed to the description of developmental language disorders. More recent attempts to delineate subtypes are discussed and commonalities between different models are noted. The last section taking, as a starting point, the Rapin and Allen classification, describes a range of developmental disorders using case illustrations drawn from the authors' clinical experience as examples.

This chapter will examine some of the clinical subtypes of developmental language disorder as they are presented in the literature and discuss their relationship to the nature of language disorders as described in Chapter 4. Some of the early attempts at differentiation have been indicated in Chapter 1 together with reasons for making such attempts. As was stated in that chapter, the first simple divisions into expressive and receptive language disorders are now seen to be unsatisfactory for such a division cannot adequately take into account interrelationship of levels which form a part of the language processing model. Nevertheless, the clinical subtypes now emerging do tend to follow a receptive–expressive, or input–output, pattern, but the former dichotomy is replaced by a recognition of the effect one has on the other. Additionally, there is no longer a discrete emphasis on exclusivity of types of language disorder, for as many studies suggest the boundaries are 'fuzzy'.

In the field of acquired aphasia, or the breakdown of language in adults, the differentiation of clinical subtypes has been very helpful to the propagation of clinical techniques. They have generated clear methodologies by which patients can be diagnosed, treated and their progress be appraised. They have contributed to the exchange of information both between disciplines and between international professional bodies because they have provided a framework in which exchanges can take place. Their limitations arise from too strict an adherence to the model so that there is sometimes a tendency to fit all patterns into the framework. Caramazza and Zurif (1978) explored this aspect and concluded that there is no simple or direct relationship between developmental and acquired disorders. However, even though the models generating the subtypes and methodologies may be superseded, the stimulus towards experiment and thought given by the clear differentiation of subtypes has undoubtedly advanced remedial procedures. We are not yet at the point in the developmental field where a working dialogue can easily be created among professionals because of the subtype structure. It seems that language in dissolution lends itself more easily to analysis than does language in development. Also we can still obtain clearer information from the damaged brain than from the developing one when subjected to neurological investigation. With the increasing sophistication of imaging techniques and growing evidence from cerebral blood flow studies there is the likelihood that increased knowledge will accrue. Geschwind has pointed out in a number of different papers that 'brains which show no pathology in the usual sense of the term may yet deviate from the normal'. We know that when language users suffer cerebral damage, their language tends to break down in certain ways. We cannot be so sure of the manner in which language is actually acquired. It has yet to be convincingly demonstrated that language-disordered children process language in a different manner from normal children and that the differences in processing are associated with particular types of language disorder. Neither is there overwhelming evidence to suggest that specific impairments in processing lead to specific subtypes of language disorder. However, these are hypotheses we must pursue as we try to make sense of what we find in our clinical population. If we combine these hypotheses and enlarge them to include language processing which is inefficient, rather than aberrant, we can keep some flexibility while continuing to search for clarity.

Undoubtedly there are parallels between acquired and developmental language pathology; verbal auditory agnosia, for example, bears some similarity to Wernicke's aphasia. But impairment of development and breakdown of function need to be seen against very different backgrounds. In the case of an adult with an acquired disorder, the breakdown is likely to occur in the context of a previously normal functioning linguistic system so that remnants of this will still be evident in varying degrees. Where language impairment is developmental there is no such background of experience. Different too will be the progress of the condition. Natural processes of maturation will exert influence on developing language however impaired, so that the pattern of deficit may then change. The adult, on the other hand, may through disease be subject to what Critchley has so eloquently termed 'the drift and dissolution of language'.

Age of emergence

When considering clinical subtypes we need therefore to take into consideration the age at which they emerge and their constancy over time. Language delay may herald difficulties with linguistic and behavioural features which only become apparent later. Children who show persistent delay in both comprehension and expression have a poorer prognosis than those whose difficulties are centred in one aspect or the other (Silva and Ferguson, 1980). This is probably because of the strong association between broad language delay and severe learning difficulties. Bishop and Edmundson (1987a) found that isolated linguistic impairments in young children carried a better prognosis than did more pervasive ones. Stark, Mellits and Tallal (1983) suggest that some language-delayed children may with maturity show gains in the individual subskills which underpin language as well as in their ability to compensate for specific deficiencies. This view is in accord with their hypothesis that for children with specific language impairment there may be a dissociation between receptive and expressive language. Children who present with delay in all aspects of expressive language may master a degree of form and then settle into a recalcitrant pattern of phonological disability. This is illustrated by Bishop and Edmundson in a helpful 'submerged mountains' diagram in which they show that some functions, e.g. phonology, may remain affected while others to which they are related improve. The more areas of function that are involved the greater the impairment and the poorer the prognosis. The pattern of disorder will change with development, leaving only the most vulnerable elements still at risk. It follows that if many elements are involved, even shifts in the pattern will leave the child without an adequate basis for language learning. The fact that children with developmental disorders of language do show shifts in pattern over time is emphasised by Rapin and Allen (1983) as they present their own delineation of syndromes of developmental language disorder. These authors base their findings upon data derived from preschool children studied longitudinally, school-aged children with severe developmental language disorders and children from a special preschool nursery who presented with a variety of developmental disorders. There appears to be a consensus of opinion among investigators that clinical subtypes or patterns of impairment should not be described before around 3 years of age. Aram and Nation (1975) projected their patterns of behaviour from a population of between 3;2 and 6;11 years. Wolfus, Moscovitch and Kinsbourne (1980) used a sample with age range from 4;2 to 7;5 years. Wilson and Risucci (1986) established their clinical classification from a sample with an age range of 3;0–5;1 years.

If subgroups or clinical subtypes are to include children as young as 3;0 years, it is quite reasonable to suppose that there will be a shift in pattern over time. It would be rather surprising if there were not. The necessity for the exercise of classifying at such an early age may then be questioned. The broad classification offered by Bloom and Lahey in which the child's language behaviour is deemed to represent disorders of form, content and use has a good deal to recommend it. This was first described in the authors' 1978 text and came as a very welcome, practical way of looking at language breakdown or maldevelopment (Bloom and Lahey, 1978). It cut across the medical models which had previously dominated the field, but was simpler and more immediately effective than the linguistic ones then emerging. Children with different kinds of developmental disabilities could be classified by the methods propagated by Bloom and Lahey and the broad classification could then be amplified by more detailed description of the child's language. Nevertheless, while deserving to stand as a model of useful practice, supported by considerable scholarship, the Bloom–Lahey classification has not, in itself, taken us far enough in our search to understand all the different ways in which language can fail to develop in young children who are not globally retarded, autistic or hearing impaired. A similar comment can be applied to the classification proposed by Wiig and Semel (1976). This is based on a cognitive processing model which proposes seven categories under this general heading. These are intended to describe the uses of language, but no explanation is offered as to how any interference would contribute to specific language impairment. The next wave of investigation prompted by the need for more accurate prediction and the desire for more effective remediation is now well advanced.

Patterns of deficit

Aram and Nation undertook one of the first of this new wave of investigations by studying 47 children with developmental language disorders. Their object was to provide data on an aetiologically heterogeneous sample. Such data could then be used to group children together for classification purposes and to show differential patterns of language. The investigation employed a battery of 14 language tasks taken from standardised tests. Six different patterns of deficit were found from the factor analysis of task scores. They are summarised in the following list:

- Ability to repeat is better than the ability to comprehend or generate language.
- There is a non-specific or general formulation–repetition deficit.
- There is general low performance across all language tasks.
- There is specific difficulty at the phonological level affecting comprehension, formulation and repetition.
- Comprehension is impaired in relation to other language skills.
- There is formulation–repetition deficit with adequate comprehension.

Hearing loss was a disqualification for inclusion in the study, but the authors did not, as later reseachers have done, stipulate that overall intelligence must be within normal limits. They did not consider the data then available justified special IQ criteria for inclusion. When they reviewed 20 of their original sample (Aram and Nation, 1980), they found that 20% had WISC scores in the mentally handicapped range and were being educated in special classrooms for such pupils. Of the remaining number, 69% needed special tutoring and grade replacements at some time. The grade replacements included transfer to a learning disabilities class. In their chart review, Aram and Nation found that 40% of their subjects continued to present with language or articulatory disorders, reading and spelling difficulties.

Other points arising from these important studies will be considered elsewhere in the text since the focus of this chapter is on clinical subtypes. Looking at their original groups, the authors found that the profiles of children in group 1 had remained relatively static. The next group with pattern 2 deficit were described as 'shifters' with marked changes in strengths and weaknesses. Two-thirds of the pupils in this group were experiencing academic problems. The group 3 children had all continued to show language difficulties and their overall academic level had made them highly represented among those being educated in classes for the mentally handicapped. When children who had been placed in the learning disabilities class were examined, it was found that though their profiles had shifted, they did not show any one single language pattern. The 1980 follow-up study looked at less than half the original sample from which the patterns or subgroups were derived and the main purpose of the study was to examine the relationship between preschool language disorders and academic difficulties. The inability to substantiate the constancy of the original patterns across time is therefore not surprising. A further follow-up published in 1984 (Aram, Ekelman and Nation, 1984) is based on individual assessment and does not consider group pattern data. In their original paper Aram and Nation (1975) state that they have found the classification by differential deficits to be meaningful and clinically useful to themselves, but more widespread application would have to be made before the six patterns could be established. If the patterns proved to be demonstrable only in the original population, it could be that they were associated with the battery of tests used (see Chapter 6).

Developmental language disorder syndromes

This section will consider some of the clinical studies which have been published within the last 10 years (i.e. since 1980) in which the authors have attempted to identify specific subgroups of disorder. At the time of writing, research is continuing with the intention of clarifying the classifications and of thereby indicating strategies for remediation. Four main studies will be described and areas of commonality will be considered. From the standpoint of our own clinical experience through case studies, we will discuss the relationship between some of the subgroups and the language processing model described in Chapter 4.

Rapin and Allen (1983) start from a medical viewpoint by heading their chapter 'Nosological conditions'. 'Nosology' is a medical term which refers to the process of delineating a disease entity. Their data are, however, derived from a number of different sources: clinical data from the charts of approximately 100 children referred for neuropaediatric consultation with the chief complaint of delayed or deviant speech; videotape recordings from approximately 20 preschool children obtained over a 1–3 year period: formal analysis of the language of 20 school-aged children with severe developmental language disorders; longitudinal studies of children enrolled in a therapeutic nursery, age range 3–5 years, with a variety of disturbances including autism. The authors state that although the Aram and Nation study was limited to standardised tasks, resemblances can be found between their patterns and some of the syndromes derived independently by them from their study of children's performance under naturalistic conditions. Rapin and Allen state that their own syndromes should not be regarded as exhaustive. Their main purpose is to indicate that there is no one diagnosis. Their subjects were grouped according to the most salient characteristics of their expressive language, interactive behaviour and apparent comprehension. The syndromes were then defined by determining which language features were impaired, intact or variable within each subgroup. The authors also challenge the view that language disorders can only be postulated in the presence or near-presence of normal intelligence. They emphasise that the IQ is useful for making distinctions and predictions among normal children, but is much less meaningful when applied to handicapped children whose performance across tests is uneven. They believe that an attempt to study language disorder by looking for a 'pure' form, i.e. one that is not contaminated by low IQ means that investigators will not be considering the majority of children seen by clinicians. Language disorders are also to be found in children with other manifestations of brain dysfunction. This supports the position taken by Aram and Nation. However, Rapin and Allen by moving away from standardised tests make it less likely that they will come up with a group of children with overall low functioning such as that found by Aram and Nation and also by Silva.

The syndromes are described in 1983 under the following headings.

Phonosyntactic syndrome

This is stated to be the most prevalent of the syndromes. It is seen by the authors as showing features similar to the expressive disorders described by Morley (1972) and T.T.S. Ingram (1959). The principal impairments are in the phonological and morphosyntactic systems. Disturbances may include severely limited use of function words and inflections of nouns and verbs as well as severe limitations of syntactic relations expressed within a single utterance. Many of these children have other signs of neurological dysfunction, the most prevalent being oromotor dysfunction. However, the fact that the group includes those whose phonological skills are better in repetition than in spontaneous utterance suggests that the deficit lies in motor programming rather than in motor production. Rapin and Allen discuss the possible neurological correlates, which could be attributable to prefrontal pathology which encroaches on the motor cortex or possibly to some cortical connections. Where comprehension is also defective, the temporal or temporoparietal areas may be suspect.

Severe expressive syndrome with good comprehension

These children are described as being mute or virtually unintelligible. Their comprehension is good and may be demonstrated through some kind of alternative communication system. The neurological basis is not clear.

Verbal auditory agnosia

Since the block is in the input processing, these children have no comprehension of speech. While they can be distinguished from autistic children by other than language behaviour, e.g. good eye contact, they may develop sufficiently severe secondary symptoms to make the differential diagnosis difficult. This is the one group which appears to have been constantly cited throughout the history of language classification. It is virtually identical to that described by Worster-Drought and Allen in 1930 and subsequently elaborated in a series of publications and also by Eisenson in 1968. The basis for the condition is stated by Rapin and Allen to be bilateral temporal lobe pathology.

Mute autistic syndrome

These are stated to be the children with the most profound and usually irreversible syndrome of developmental language disorder. They are impaired in oral language and in symbolic function in general. They fail to make use of any method of communication. The neurological basis is unknown.

Autistic syndrome with echolalia

These children are characterised by their ability to repeat fairly long sequences of well-formed utterances heard previously. Some become hyperlexic. Both echolalia and hyperlexia are suggestive of deficient semantic processing of discourse. From the neurological point of view, it is suggested that there must be some intact pathways between areas concerned with phonological reception (primary auditory cortex) and production (primary motor cortex) and also between visual perception and the main language areas of the cortex.

Semantic–pragmatic syndrome without autism

These children have fluent expressive language, but it is not really communicative. Comprehension of discourse is impaired though short units may be understood. Echolalia may be present. The syndrome has been observed in children with hydrocephalus, but may also be present in children without other evidence of brain dysfunction. These children's use of social or stereotyped utterances lacking in content or originality has led to the term 'cocktail party syndrome' (Tew, 1979). In hydrocephalic children, the semantic–pragmatic syndrome may accompany cognitive impairment. The site of major pathology is the subcortical white matter affecting intrahemispherical pathways.

Syntactic–pragmatic syndrome

The characteristics of this syndrome are grossly impaired syntax and severely limited pragmatic use of language. Comprehension of connected discourse is also impaired as are the demands of interpersonal conversation. Rapin and Allen are unable to speculate as to the neurological basis for this disorder which they have found to be extremely rare. They state that this was the only group of children whose syntax was severely affected but whose phonology was normal or near normal.

In their presentation in 1987, Rapin and Allen described their subtypes with some modifications. These were:

- Verbal auditory agnosia or word deafness: this description remains unchanged.
- Verbal dyspraxia: this would now appear to correspond to one group of the severe expressive syndrome.
- Phonological programming deficit syndrome: the utterance is more fluent than for verbal dyspraxia, but intelligibility is poor or very poor. This group would make up the remainder of those originally classified under the severe expressive syndrome.
- Phonological–syntactic syndrome: description unchanged.
- Lexical–syntactic deficit syndrome: these children usually begin to speak late but with normal phonology. They show severe word retrieval deficit and have difficulty in formulating connected language.
- Semantic–pragmatic deficit syndrome: description unchanged.

The authors did not include the autistic syndromes in this 1987 classification which related to clinical subtypes in language-disordered and autistic children. References were made to the syndromes as they presented in autism. It is of interest that autistic syndromes were included in the original classification for they are not always noted in studies of developmental language disorders; indeed many specifically exclude them, together with hearing loss and cognitive impairment. Other authors, e.g. Rutter, have also shown interest in the way the populations meet and diverge. (See Boucher (1976) and, more recently, Bishop (1989) for an overview of autism and language disorder.)

Rapin and Allen are currently engaged in a multidisciplinary, multicentre study which has as its goals:

● To identify the most powerful measures which will discriminate developmental language disorders from autism spectrum disorders and from mental deficiency in preschool children.
● To identify behaviourally defined empirically validated subtypes within developmental language disorder and autism spectrum disorder.

Some preliminary results are reported in the 1987 paper. In discussing their categories, the authors state that the full range of variability within each is not yet known. They also emphasise that the fact that boundaries to the condition are frequently blurred does not mean that the syndromes are invalid.

Bishop and Rosenbloom (1987) affirm several of the categories offered by Rapin and Allen and by doing so in a large multidisciplinary text have increased the likelihood of the categories being generally accepted. They agree with the subtype phonological–syntactic syndrome and identify it as relating to specific problems with language form.

With regard to semantic–pragmatic syndrome Bishop and Rosenbloom prefer the term 'disorder' to 'syndrome' for this condition since they believe that a loosely associated set of behaviours relating to language use and content is being described. These they regard as shading into autism at one extreme and normality at the other. They suggest that research studies into these disorders are urgently needed and offer a set of hypotheses in the form of comments. Clinical descriptions are offered in an attempt to share knowledge about these children in whom there is considerable current interest. This interest has been growing since the 1970s when case reports and clinical descriptions of language-disordered children started to be more widely circulated. It combined with the upsurge of interest in pragmatic function. Bloom and Lahey were among the first to suggest ways in which to look at children whose problems did not extend to language form. There is also an interesting territorial development both in the USA and in the UK with regard to disorders of content and function. If semantic–pragmatic disorder is accepted as a language problem, the child will need the care of language therapists; if it is part of an autistic syndrome, there is less likelihood of the speech–language pathologist–therapist becoming involved. Professions do therefore have a vested interest in establishing the precise nature of abnormal language behaviour, but this must not be allowed to detract from the interests of the child.

Wilson and Risucci (1986) refer to the Rapin–Allen model as being clinically derived and imply that its acceptance must await more hard data. They also point out that the Aram and Nation study failed to address issues of either internal or external validity (a point recognised by the authors in their statement that widespread substantiation would be necessary before the patterns could be accepted). Wilson and Risucci are also critical of another study (Wolfus, Moscovitch and Kinsbourne, 1980) which delineated two subgroups of developmental language disorders on the basis of a variety of neuropsychological and linguistic measures. Wolfus, Moscovitch and Kinsbourne attempted to divide their developmentally language-impaired children into subgroups. They considered one group with syntactic and/or semantic deficit with a view to dividing them into those with deficits in syntax production and those with syntax production and comprehension deficits. It was also proposed to consider whether the broad group could be divided in another way, namely into one group which was semantically normal and another which was semantically impaired. Differences in expressive phonology which could be related to different types of language impairment were also to be investigated. A third aim was to determine whether auditory–perceptual deficits would account for language impairment. This was a topic highly current in the late 1970s and early 1980s largely due to the continuing work of Tallal which has been cited previously. Locke's (1980) overview of auditory perceptual assessments is discussed in Chapter 6. The perceptual–cognitive–linguistic battery employed by Wolfus, Moscovitch and Kinsbourne did succeed in achieving some differentiations between groups. Sample size was 19 and the children who had a mean age of 5;7 years had been diagnosed by speech pathologists as being language disordered. The children were all within the normal range on tests of intelligence. In summary, they found no support for an auditory perceptual basis for language impairments. They found two groups represented within their sample:

1. An expressive group characterised by deficits in the production of syntax and phonology.
2. A group of expressive–receptive impairment characterised by deficits in phonological discrimination, digit span and semantic ability as well as showing global syntactic impairment.

The Wilson–Risucci model (1986) was developed to avoid the

inadequacies which those authors considered to be associated with studies relying only on clinical inference. The typology they propose stems from an assessment model which demands the incorporation of psychometric and clinical–observational data. Their classification is based on a branching model rather than on a fixed battery. Thus the investigator can be guided to further investigations and probings by the child's pattern of response. This follows the thinking of those who regard classification as hypothesis testing rather than as an allocation to clinically or theoretically constructed groups. Five groups were hypothesised by the authors on the basis of:

● Consensus among five clinical neuropsychologists.
● Language pathologists' reports.
● Comparison with subgroups defined by a cluster analytical approach.
● Comparison among subgroups on variables not used for classification.

Results are discussed with relation to a number of important issues and a helpful chart is generated showing commonalities with the typologies of Aram and Nation, and Rapin and Allen upon which we will draw. Wilson and Risucci have in train a number of studies relating to stability, remediation, reading prediction and brain behaviour. They also suggest that indications may be confirmed which will show that the same subtypes in addition to others will be found in further clinical populations including cerebral palsy, hydrocephalus, the Gilles de la Tourette syndrome and learning disabilities.

The 1986 paper by Wilson and Risucci arises from earlier studies (Wilson, 1979, 1981) which are not easily available in the UK and this may explain why the work is rarely cited by British speech therapists. The constructs used within their tests are, however, familiar as are most of the language and cognitive tests through which they are demonstrated. The constructs are auditory perception, discrimination and cognition (related to levels of auditory semantic comprehension), auditory memory and retrieval, and visual discrimination, visual spatial, visual cognition and visual memory. These constructs as identified in particular combinations give each case its individual profile. The database is very different from that used in other studies cited and the authors point out that it is differences of databases which limit the extent to which commonalities may be inferred.

Wilson and Risucci arrive at these neuropsychological constructs through an assessment procedure in which they employ a number of subtests taken from:

● Illinois Test of Psycholinguistic Abilities (Kirk, McCarthy and Kirk, 1968).
● Goldman–Fristoe–Woodcock Test of Auditory Discrimination (Goldman, Fristoe and Woodcock, 1970).

- Wechsler Preschool and Primary Scales of Intelligence (Wechsler, 1967).
- McCarthy Scales of Children's Abilities (McCarthy, 1970).
- Hiskey–Nebraska Test of Learning Aptitude (Hiskey, 1966).
- Pictorial Test of Intelligence (French, 1964).

Similarities and divergences

Our discussion of these clinical subtypes based on our own clinical experience will focus on the Rapin and Allen model while making cross-reference to the other models described above. This does not mean that we are limited by these subtypes and indeed in some cases additional information is deemed appropriate. Table 5.1 summarises the correspondence between the terminologies employed by all these authors.

Table 5.1 Commonalities of language disorder subtypes

Rapin and Allen (1987)	Aram and Nation (1975)	Wolfus, Moscovitch and Kinsbourne (1980)	Wilson and Risucci (1986)
Verbal auditory agnosia	Generalised low performance	Comprehension + syntactic production	Global disorder
Semantic–pragmatic disorder deficit	Repetition better than comprehension	Comprehension disorder	Auditory–semantic comprehension disorder
Verbal dyspraxia	Syntactic and speech programming disorder	Syntactic production difficulty	No deficits
Phonological–syntactic disorder	Non-specific formulation repetition deficit	Syntactic production difficulty	Auditory–semantic comprehension + visual ST memory disorder
Lexical–syntactic deficit	—	Syntactic production difficulty	Expressive disorder

Verbal auditory agnosia

This is the one condition which has great consistency throughout the literature. It represents an extreme in severity of disorder and in very severe cases prognosis for development of spoken language is poor. Very severe cases are comparatively rare. Superficially these children may appear to be deaf and indeed this misdiagnosis has sometimes been made. This is understandable for characteristically they show little response to auditory stimuli whether linguistic or environmental. Extensive and in-depth assessment of hearing including brain stem evoked response audiometry tends to show that there is a response to pure tone so that peripherally, the acoustic signal is received. It would seem that the impairment lies further upstream in the central nervous system, possibly in the association auditory cortex which as we have seen is concerned with the refinement, recognition and synthesis of incoming signals. Interestingly, despite very thorough early audiological investigation, some of the children have later been found to have varying degrees of sensorineural deafness. How this comes about is a matter of speculation. It has been suggested that as a sort of defence mechanism against the babble of meaningless noise, morphological changes take place within the auditory pathway.

The main difficulty therefore is one of decoding spoken language and as a consequence encoding is also severely affected. Referring to the linguistic model of language processing, there is no possibility of extrapolation and matching from the lexical store for there has been no opportunity to acquire such a store. In other words there is nothing on which language rules can operate.

Behaviourally, particularly in the early stages, the children appear to be emotionally stable and they relate well to other people. Eisenson (1986) endorses this view. It appears as though the complete cut-off of meaningful sound cocoons them and acts as a sort of protective cover against the frustration experienced by children with predominantly production difficulties who are more aware of their limitations. The ability to form good relationships is one of the important aspects which differentiates them from autistic children.

It is obviously very difficult to determine levels of intelligence. Eisenson (1985) maintains that in this condition which he calls developmental aphasia and equates with verbal auditory agnosia and congenital auditory imperception, intelligence is adequate when measured on non-verbal scales. Our own experience based on a limited number of cases would endorse this view and we see it as representing one of the differential features between mental handicap and auditory agnosia. Some children show good ability for symbolic play without of course any verbal interaction. They show a capacity for sustained attention in such activities. These points are best illustrated by reference to the case of a boy aged 4;9 years when first seen at a children's assessment centre.

> Y. was the second child of Polish parents. The father was an agricultural worker in a very rural part of the British Isles. Birth history was normal as was subsequent motor development. He was described, however, as a very quiet baby who did not babble very much. Hearing was assessed and he was admitted to the Centre wearing two hearing aids. Subsequent testing in a neuro-audiological department elicited normal response to pure tones, so the hearing aids were removed.

He presented as an attractive flaxen haired little boy who if anything was disinhibited in his response to strangers in that he ran to them arms outstretched with a welcoming smile.

He was seen by a clinical psychologist and the Leiter International Performance Scale (Arthur, 1952) was administered. This is a measure which is designed for non-verbal children. On this he performed at low normal level as he also did on the Merrill Palmer tests.

Perceptual testing revealed a gross inability to cross-modally code information. For example, when shown three pictures, a bell, a drum and a shaker he could match the objects to the correct picture in the presence of the object as it was rung, banged or shaken. When the same noise was made behind a screen he was completely unable to identify it with the picture. As well as failure on auditory–visual input there was a similar response on haptic to visual perception. That is to say he could not match shape to pictures or to models by feel. This was particularly unfortunate as it offered little prospect of his acquiring a sign language.

He had no recognisable expressive language, but during play he would emit a continuous noise produced by vibration of his lips. This must have afforded some tactile–kinaesthetic pleasure. The warbling noise varied in length and intonation: sometimes long and high pitched and sometimes staccato. It did not appear to have any communicative function, but was an accompaniment to activity. Attempts at improving awareness of sound met with disappointing results. Obviously this case represents one of the most severe manifestations of the syndrome. He was eventually transferred to a special school for children with severe learning disability. This was in the days before widespread use of computer-based learning. It would have been interesting to have seen how much progress might have been made on a purely visual programme.

A minimally less daunting case was J. who was 4;3 years when first seen:

He was able to respond to environmental sound, but not to spoken language. Cognitive ability was assessed at low average. Hearing was normal. J. had no recognisable spoken language and unlike Y. he was not outgoing, though his severe disability was not reflected in behavioural problems. Cross-modal testing revealed a similar inability to relate visual to auditory input but he was able to link haptic and visual stimuli.

Initially therapy concentrated on linking sound and vision through mirror work whereby the psychologist or therapist modelled noises and he attempted to copy them. This met with little success and it was obvious that the method was the cause of increasing frustration. It was therefore decided to teach a very simple sign language based on the shapes which he was able to recognise. The work started initially with three shapes: a circle representing mother, a square representing himself and a triangle which signified food, the last chosen for reasons of high motivation. At a very basic level he was therefore taught to 'ask mother for food'; successful sequencing of these symbols brought a reward. The basic language was gradually elaborated, but unfortunately the eventual outcome is not known. It is possible that he would have been a good candidate for one of the systems of alternative communication which were then in their infancy.

Such cases to some extent resemble Morley's 1973 study of Sally, the main differences being that Sally had a confirmed hearing loss from the outset and that she was eventually able to acquire spoken language although this was limited by comprehension difficulties. There is also a similarity in the changed states of her peripheral hearing. This deteriorated over the years. Most of the studies rely on single cases because of their rarity. Ward and Kellett (1982) reported on eight children who suffered auditory imperception. There was some evidence of hearing loss and/or abnormal response to sound throughout the group. These authors also identified a further group as having comprehension deficits without auditory imperception. On language measures (Reynell Developmental Language Scales, RDLS, Reynell, 1977) both groups showed similarity and following intervention both showed similar gains – 15 months and 13 months respectively. The differentiating feature between the two groups lay in their response to sound. This suggests two possibilities, the first that the group designated auditory agnosia may be further divided into a subcategory in which the comprehension problems stem from other causes. The second possibility is that the 'comprehension only' group represents an interface between auditory imperception and syntactic–phonological deficit. This study does not provide data on other aspects of perception but it may well be that integrative aspects were impaired in the comprehension group. In relation to age, of the 16 children in the two groups, 8 were under 3 years when first assessed and 1 was under 4 years. Reference has been made to the difficulties faced in subtyping children before the age of 3 years and in this study follow-up data would be of considerable interest.

In terms of the Wilson and Risucci model, the comprehension group would fall into the expressive and/or receptive group. They would show impairment on auditory association and auditory reception (ITPA) and on visual reception and visual association (ITPA). These findings lend support to the hypothesis that the deficits have their origins in the angular gyrus area of the cerebral cortex which as we have seen is a region of late myelination. In terms of the information-processing model, the subgroup would show impairment at the level of semantic memory.

Semantic–pragmatic group

Although in their 1987 classification Rapin and Allen place this at the end, probably in relation to their subsequent discussion of autism, if as has been indicated, pragmatic aspects of language need to be considered at a very early stage because they are closely interwoven with semantic features, it seems appropriate to consider this subtype as following on from receptive disorders. Children with this type of disorder have been noted and described for a number of years under various labels. Reynell (1969) refers to them as 'non-creative speakers'. In other references they have been labelled as having elaborated echoic behaviour and some workers have identified the condition as being synonymous with the language deficits of autism (see correspondence in the *College of Speech Therapists Bulletin*, February and May 1988). Rapin and Allen, however, regard it as a subtype which may be a feature of autistic language, but that is not tantamount to stating that all children with this type of deficit are autistic.

Characteristically, these children are superfluent to the point of being garrulous and superficially they seem to communicate satisfactorily. However, it soon becomes apparent that the content of their language is inappropriate. They do not participate in dyadic interchange, but tend to use their listeners as a sort of spring board from which to take off on their own bizarre linguistic route. When asked questions, they will often respond by echoing the question. The following 'conversation' typifies this (where M is the child and T the therapist):

> M: He kicked me.
> T: Who kicked you?
> M: No. I don't want them
> T: Are you going home tomorrow?
> M: No.
> T: Are you going home to Mummy?
> M: Yes, No Mummy.
>   want to see Daddy
>   no Daddy
>   no sister
> T: Have you got a little girl?
> M: Yes I can't have it
>   You can't have it
>   Yes I can
>   It's trapped
>   It's no sticks
>   Hers pushed off

This exchange took place while M. was hammering a peg board and deemed to bear absolutely no relation to the activity.

In this case syntax is reasonably competent and his phonology including prosody reflects environmental dialect.

The obvious abnormalities lie in pragmatic–semantic fields. Pragmatically there is little attempt to adapt to the listener's needs, as for example, by responding to the questions. Initiation of topic may take place, but this is neither maintained nor followed through. Therefore the interchange is non-contextual.

There is no evidence of turn-taking and therefore it seems as though the therapist is in fact interrupting a particular train of the child's own utterance. This may have been so, for in response to further questions he suddenly said 'Shut up!', but this was followed over and over again like some private mantra by a repetition of this utterance.

Semantic aspects of communication appear to be by-passed for these utterances do not bear any relationship to the topic or the situation in which the child is operating. It can be concluded that perceptually the message is received, but that there is some failure between perceptual input and semantic–conceptual memory so that the input is encoded without reference to meaning.

Another child whose language could be interpreted with hindsight as being typical of semantic–pragmatic disorder was F:

> He was aged 4;6 years when first seen. He was the youngest of three boys, the other two having no history of language disorder. Birth was normal at full term, but there was a delay of circa 5 minutes in establishing respiration.
>
> Information supplied by the referring speech therapist reported no feeding or swallowing difficulties. Onset of speech was delayed and he was reported not to use sounds with meaning until after 2 years. He produced odd words just before his third birthday. By the age 4;0 years there was a sudden spurt and within a few months he was said to be using fully intelligible complex sentences, including question forms. There were some word reversals when seen at the assessment centre, language was fluent and well developed in structure, but content was inappropriate. There were a few immature phonological features. Dyadic communication was largely echoic, but normal language was heard when he was re-enacting fantasies. Examples of inappropriate content taken from recordings made at the time include:
>
> Mother: We saw Lorraine
> F: Yes its raining (it wasn't) Put up the Barricades
> M: What happened last night?
> F: Happened last night

> M: You fell out of bed didn't you?
>
> F: Yes you fell out of bed.

Receptive language was limited. He had difficulty in following complex commands. He could not match pictures, objects or animals. Concepts of colour, size or number were not developed.

The psychologist reported that on the Griffiths Developmental Scale he scored at the 5;0 year level on performance tasks. In the hearing and speech section he was down to 3;0 and 4;0 and managed only a few items. He was estimated to be a boy of normal intelligence on tests that did not require complex comprehension. Beyond simple questions his language broke down and became echoic.

It appears that F. has a poorly developed conceptual system. He perceives language and is able to retain a certain amount of linguistic information. What one hears seems to be an elaborated echoic language which has by-passed semantic levels. Obviously pragmatic features are deficient, but one would tend to regard these as the outcome of the main semantic failure.

Rapin and Allen note that this condition bears some resemblance to acquired transcortical sensory aphasia which is a fluent form resulting from damage to the area adjacent to the supramarginal gyrus. Aram and Nation in their classification acknowledge this condition by reference to an ability for repetition which can be a marked feature.

Verbal dyspraxias

In placing this syndrome next in the sequence of processing, we are undoubtedly entering a minefield of controversy. The areas of dispute lie mainly in relation to the following:

- Phonological *vs* phonetic.
- Intrinsic syntactic problems *vs* those arising as an outcome of articulatory constraints.
- Intrinsic prosodic problems *vs* those arising as an outcome of articulatory constraints.

Perhaps it may be most fruitful to begin by defining what we construe to be the nature of developmental dyspraxia. We consider it to be an impairment in the selection, planning and programming of linguistic and of motor schemata for production of language.

There is no evidence of peripheral motor impairment and within the limits of current methods of assessment of verbal comprehension there does not appear to be any deficit at this level. The inclusion of 'selection' as one of the features betokens the possibility of an impairment which may have its origins in higher cortical function. Referring back to the processing model based on Garrett (1980), it will be seen that, at a fairly early stage, retrieval of phonological representations of content words takes place. These are fitted into the linguistic frame. This operation is closely followed by the generation of the framework for function words. Evidence from slips of the tongue data in relation to normal speakers demonstrates that mis-selection can occur very early on in the planning programme. Boomer and Laver (1968) differentiate between slips which indicate a semantic mismatch and those where phonological elements are involved. In the former case there is competition between two semantically associated words /I haven't the sleast idea→slightest and least/, and in the latter there is a sequencing error /plincipal frute→principal flute (attributed to Radio 3)/. This last example shows a transposition of second element cluster. Similar types of realisations have been documented in children with developmental disorders, e.g. /I like treacle fot fot toffee/.

Crary (1984) considers that developmental verbal dyspraxia (DVD) is a more linguistically encompassing disorder than the adult counterpart. It is unlikely that it is a unitary disorder and undoubtedly, in some respects, it is difficult to distinguish from the phonological–syntactic disorder described by Rapin and Allen. It may be a matter of degree, for these authors appear to delineate a very severe form in which the child may be virtually mute.

Panagos and Bobkoff (1984) also support the view that the disorder originates in higher linguistic programming; in fact they designate it as a cognitive–linguistic disorder. They reject the idea that it is confined to the phonological level and demonstrate convincingly that because of the interactive nature of encoding, which will be discussed further in Chapter 6, pragmatic, semantic and syntactic aspects are involved. A 'pure motor' theory could not allow for this and therefore a motor–cognitive model is accepted. This accords with the views expressed and with the model discussed in the chapter on the nature of language processing. We consider this view to reflect our own clinical findings. It has been noted, for example, in a pilot study carried out by Edwards (1982) that non-segmental aspects of language are adversely affected. In tasks involving change of stress which also alter speaker's intention, since English is a stress timed language, these children are unable to signal change of stress with change of meaning. Stress tends to be equal and even. Syntax suffers under the influence of increased complication of phonological patterns and this most commonly involves the deletion of function words: 'she started on her way home' 'she go home'

Crary in his study of 25 children was able to delineate a hierarchy of difficulty at phonological level. Dominant errors were syntagmatic in nature i.e. they included omissions (dominating the most severe cases), cluster reductions, voicing errors, metathesis and assimilation. Less severe cases included more paradigmatic errors, i.e. substitution. These were more apparent in phrase repetition than in word repetition. Edwards' 1982 sample manifested all these features, although a preponderance of omissions did not emerge. Metathesis, assimilation and voicing errors were dominant.

It has been pointed out that the phonological errors made by dyspraxic children differ from those associated with maturational delay. In the case of cluster reduction, for example, the delay process pattern in /st-/ clusters would be deletion of the fricative; the dyspraxic child may reduce by omitting the second element of the cluster: /stocking>socking/. Similarly voicing errors may be voiced>voiceless or voiceless>voiced, e.g. paper>bader and duck>tuck.

This last example illustrates the inconsistency which has been described in a number of studies as a salient feature.

Similar errors are frequently apparent in written work and many of these children experience difficulty with reading.

Associated motor errors have been noted. The word 'associated' is used advisedly for a direct cause—effect explanation is not tenable. Current neurophysiology (e.g. Netsell, 1986) regards motor programming of movement as being distinct from movement for speech. For this reason, remediation which concentrates on exercise of articulatory organs other than in the context of speech is not likely to be fruitful.

Eleven out of the 13 children in the Edwards' pilot study had concomitant movement impairment. This tendency has led to such children being described as clumsy (Walton, Ellis and Court, 1962; Gubbay, 1975; Gordon and McKinlay, 1980). Their impairment relates to both gross and fine motor activities — hopping, kicking, throwing, threading etc. Diadochokinetic movement is also affected as noted by Yoss and Darley (1974) who regarded this as one of the 'soft' neurological signs in their sample. In a replication of this study (Williams, Ingham and Rosenthal, 1981), this was the only factor of similarity. Aetiology is unclear but there are indications, in some cases, of damage or disorder in the posterior temporal region. Rapin and Allen cite a number of blood flow studies and Crary draws upon evidence from limited post-mortem findings.

Aram and Nation's studies confirm many of the features described above. Because of the nature of their assessment protocol, this particular constellation was not revealed in the Wilson and Risucci work and they note that had it not included information from clinical observation, disorders of spoken language would not have been observed.

Phonological—syntactic disorder

Rapin and Allen have subdivided their original classification into phonological—programming deficit syndrome and phonological—syntactic syndrome. The former subgroup seems to be a bridge between verbal dyspraxia and the latter subtype. Differences appear to relate mainly to degree of severity. The phonological–syntactic syndrome also in many ways resembles the features of verbal dyspraxia as described here, but Rapin and Allen differentiate it in noting that it is combined with comprehension deficits although these are not as severe as the production disorder. They draw parallels between this condition and Broca's aphasia citing, as evidence, omission of word endings and function words. Bishop and Rosenbloom (1987) question this comparison with evidence that lesions of Broca's area do not always result in this type of aphasia and conversely it is found where there are no lesions in that area. This argument reflects the qualifications which were made at the beginning of this chapter. Wilson and Risucci regard the disorder as being closely related to deficits in auditory–semantic comprehension and visual short-term memory; in other words they appear to regard the expressive deficit as being secondary to reception although they classify it as expressive–receptive. Chapter 7 on intervention discusses further, through case illustration, the blurred nature of difference between phonological–syntactic disorder and verbal dyspraxia.

> R. aged 4;11 when first seen conveyed information in telegraphese. Language consisted mainly of content words, and verb tense was invariably the present. A LARSP analysis [Crystal, Fletcher and Garman, 1976] showed that the majority of syntactic structures lay at stage 3 with a predominance of three element clauses: /my daddy car Nada [Granada], that buses single desker [decker]/.
>
> Auditory memory was extremely limited and on the ITPA digit repetition test he scored at the 3;3 year level. He was unable to carry out triple commands – 'go to the window, pick up the pencil and bring it to me'. Recall of the Bus Story was fragmented. Colour naming presented severe difficulties although he could match well. This may have been a word-finding difficulty (see next section). He dealt with this problem of which he was very much aware by labelling all colours as 'purple'.
>
> Phonologically, there was evidence of weak syllable deletion, cluster reduction and variability (stairs>sairs>tairs), and also metathesis (deckers>desker). Affricates were realised as fricatives.

In some ways R.'s disorder resembled that of Ruth described by Chiat and Hirson (1987). Fletcher's discussion of this paper in the same issue raises some interesting points. He considers that Ruth's reasonably good level of comprehension may have been apparent rather than real and he provides possible instances of deficit. Chiat and Hirson advance a tentative explanation for the syntactic and semantic impairment being the result of phonological constraints, but Fletcher comments that within the data there are indications of alternative explanations for this type of disorder; for example, failure at some other point in the system, lexical access or the production analogue of the syntactic parser. He draws upon his current research as evidence that such possibilities should be considered although he concedes that, because of the fact that there is at the present time a paucity of hard evidence about the nature of language processing, the Chiat and Hirson explanation may well be correct.

Lexical–syntactic deficit

Children with this deficit have predominantly word-finding problems. They are thought to be late in developing speech and are said to be rather quiet infants. There do, however, appear to be two subgroups:

1. Those who remain quiet and have a sparsity of language with difficulty in retrieving lexical items.
2. Those who have similar word-finding difficulties, but who use a variety of word fillers in an effort to retrieve words.

This second subgroup has a similar or even greater output than normally speaking children, but much of the content is empty. German has documented this disorder in a number of studies (1985, 1987). Her first study was based on work carried out by Wiig and Semel (1984) who include items for assessment of word-finding difficulty in their CELF inventory. These were confrontation naming experiments in which performance was compared with normal controls and with children with learning disabilities but without word-finding problems. Semantic classes selected were numbers, letters and colours. These were presented in both sequential and randomised form. Significant differences were found between the groups, the learning disabled/word-finding difficulty group performing particularly poorly on colour and letter naming. This was most apparent when the items were presented randomly. They also tended to take a much longer time to complete the tasks. Strategies employed to retrieve a name included a recital of colours until the correct one was 'found'. German remarks that it appeared as if the children were sifting through their semantic colour file. The second study reported in 1987 investigated word-finding difficulties in conversational situations. It was in this study that the difference noted above in relation to subgroups was observed. This confirms anecdotal clinical evidence. Word-finding deficits occurring in isolation are comparatively rare; in this respect the develop-mental condition differs from an acquired disorder where an anomic aphasia is more frequent. They do, however, appear as part of a constellation of problems. The extract cited on p.188 of the boy who circumlocuted because he was unable to retrieve the name which he knew and wanted is an example of this, for word finding was only one of his many other problems.

R. who was described in the previous section as having a predominantly phonological–syntactic deficit was also noted to have word-finding deficits. German lists 15 characteristics of this condition. An important criterion is of course the fact that the child actually *knows* the word he is seeking so that failure to produce it is clearly attributable to retrieval. Various forms of circumlocution are evident, e.g. describing by function, giving associated words, either paradigmatic or syntagmatic, use of vague words, filled pauses – 'this kind of thing, er um' etc. Use of gesture including facial grimacing, incomplete phrases and self-corrections with false starts. German's subjects were in a somewhat older age group, 7;0–12;0 years, but plainly her findings have useful implications for younger children. Children with word-finding difficulties are said to have good comprehension. Whereas the presenting problem is at word level, there is obviously some accompanying degradation of syntax. Retrieval from semantic memory is hypothesised as being the source of the deficit, but the possibility that conceptual organisation may also be a source of error needs to be considered.

Phonological disorder

Rapin and Allen do not consider this as a subtype which exists in isolation and it is certainly difficult to dissociate it from some degree of concomitant deficit involving other levels of language.

The results of assessment in the study by Edwards *et al.* (1984) lend support to this view. Of 191 children who were assessed on three measures (EAT, TACL and LARSP) only 7.3% were found to have isolated phonological/articulation deficits. The greatest number scored low on a combination of EAT and LARSP (42%) followed by all three tests (30.8%).

Table 5.2 Summary of salient deviant features in subtypes of language disorders

	Comprehension	Production			Pragmatic
		Semantic	Syntactic	Phonological	
Verbal auditory agnosia	– – –	– – –	– – –	– – –	– – –
Semantic–pragmatic	– –	– – –	–	+	– – –
Verbal dyspraxia	+	+	– –	– – –	+
Phonological–syntactic	–	+	– –	– –	+
Lexical–syntactic	+	– –	–	+	+

–, Some impairment; – –, moderate impairment; – – –, severe impairment; +, not markedly impaired.

Crystal (1987) drawing on clinical data demonstrates the interaction between segmental and non-segmental phonology and grammatical complexity. Ingram (1987) hypothesises that there is an inverse relationship between vocabulary and phonological development. It is not within the scope of this text nor is it within the competence of the authors to consider in detail the range of different types of phonological disability. Grunwell (1980a, 1981, 1982a) probably offers the most authoritative account. There is also a group of interesting discussion papers by Hewlett, Grunwell, Milroy, Harris and Cottam and Hawkins (all published in the *British Journal of Disorders of Communication*, 1985, Vol. 20).

Table 5.2 provides a summary of salient characteristics associated with each of the subtypes described above. The description of subtypes of language disorder described here is not definitive. It is also recognised that within each type, there are gradations. Clinicians will recognise certain signs within their clinical population. In order to affirm these hypotheses we now need to consider ways in which children's language may be assessed.

Chapter 6
Assessment of Language Disorders

Summary

This chapter begins by discussing the justification for assessment. This is followed by a review of different methods and the limitations and strengths of both formal and naturalistic approaches are considered. There then follows a more detailed account of current practice with regard to investigation including profiling methods. Finally, issues of accountability are addressed.

For the majority of speech therapists currently in practice, assessment is a routine step in the process of remediation. Following a preliminary interview, decisions are taken as to which measures are likely to be the most appropriate, either to confirm or negate an initial hypothesis regarding the nature of the individual's language disorder. These days therapists are able to select from a wide range of test instruments, and the temptation to run the gamut of these, particularly when no clear picture emerges, is understandable. This has not always been the case. The advent of so many tests has only happened since the early to mid-1960s. Indeed it is reported that one very eminent practitioner maintained that the only equipment a good therapist needed was a pencil and a piece of paper. For someone with vast experience and finely tuned sensitivity this may have sufficed; for lesser beings such resources seem barely adequate.

The justification for assessment

Why therefore is assessment regarded as such an intrinsic part of the therapeutic process? The main reasons may be categorised thus:

● First and possibly of paramount importance is the need to provide a description of the strengths and weaknesses of the child's linguistic system.

● To offer a prognosis.
● To attempt an explanation for the disorder – a diagnosis.
● To indicate possible methods of intervention.
● To procure comparative data from which change can be measured.
● For purposes of research.

Descriptive data

The philosophy of testing has undergone radical change in recent years. Just as at one time examinations seemed to be designed to expose ignorance rather than to reveal knowledge, so language tests appeared to be slanted towards error counts, e.g. The Templin Darley articulation test was based on such a model. Stimulus words contained a range of speech sounds in initial medial and final position and these were scored on a right–wrong count. There was no provision for an appraisal of the 'errors' (The Edinburgh Articulation Test was one of the earlier ones to include this component) and consequently indications for treatment had to be arrived at by the therapist, often on an intuitive basis.

From this practice we have moved towards a system of profiling the child's language. This entails taking a more global view so that instead of focusing solely on the prevailing difficulty, the need to consider how this may affect other aspects of communicative ability is recognised. This consideration extends to non-linguistic behaviours too, for as has been described in Chapter 1, a language disability may well have a pervasive effect in the much wider context of the child in relation to the environment. In terms of language levels too, discrete impairment is unlikely. For example, what may at first appear as a straightforward phonological problem can have implications for syntactic, prosodic and possibly semantic and pragmatic aspects too (Panagos, 1982). What we are mainly concerned with now is to try to determine the nature of the child's linguistic system.

To offer a prognosis

This presents many difficulties in so far as it is influenced (1) by unforseen variables arising in the course of therapy and (2) by our present state of knowledge.

In Chapter 3 we described some of these problems. Chief among them is to decide whether the presenting disorder constitutes a maturational delay and if so will it resolve spontaneously, or whether the child is set on course for a pattern of deviant language development which may prove intractable unless early and appropriate intervention is available. Bishop and Edmundson (1987b) have begun to address this issue as one of the aims of their longitudinal study. Their subjects were a group of 88 children whose language development was a source of concern. They were assessed on a series of language tests at ages of 3;9 and 5;5 years. Results showed a hierarchy of disorder with the outcome being least favourable for those children with the greatest number of language functions impaired. Isolated impairments such as a pure phonological disorder were more likely to resolve. It has to be said that their measurement of phonology was fairly cursory in that it relied on the percentage of consonants recorded as being correct. It may well be that within this grouping there was considerable variation depending on the pattern of deficit.

Additionally one must take into account constitutional factors within the child as well as those which impinge upon him environmentally. Wedell (1980) has described the influence of compensatory interaction on the degree of success: 'the extent to which a child is motivated to use whatever limited abilities he has determines his degree of success' (p. 16).

The need for an explanation

Possibly in terms of diagnosis this is regarded as being less important than was the case some years ago. The emphasis on explanations or diagnosis undoubtedly has its roots in the medical model from which early studies of speech pathology derived. Lund, writing in 1986, comments on 'the traditional way of conceptualising the problem, which has been to view the disorder as a pathological state' (p. 415). Closely linked to diagnosis is the question of aetiology. It is accepted that at present no cause can be ascribed in the case of many developmental disorders. Bishop and Rosenbloom (1987) in a discussion of causation underline this point and go on to speculate that many language disorders may have a multifactorial basis. Robinson (1987) was able to identify possible causative factors in the group of children he studied, but this was a highly selected group receiving special investigation because of the severity of their language disorder. In such circumstances it is therefore more straightforward to deduce causation from the results of assessment. But even so, there is a need for caution. If the types of language disorder associated with the cerebral palsies were taken as an example, it would not be helpful to assume a direct cause–effect relationship just from the physical condition. Other possibilities, both psychological and neurological, need to be taken into account. Therefore the most that may be posited is *an association* (Edwards, 1984).

In a slightly different sense, i.e. non-aetiological, explanations are important. The information obtained from the various assessments, cognitive as well as linguistic, is somewhat akin to the clues of a crossword puzzle. From each one a meaning must be derived and this, in turn, must relate to the sum total of data so that in the end a composite pattern emerges. Our new-found enthusiasm for descriptive statements should not beguile us into thinking that this is sufficient. We also need to try to discover how the child's linguistic system is operating and why it is thus.

To indicate possible methods of intervention

This is a self-evident fact. The idea of embarking upon therapy on an *ad hoc* basis would nowadays find little favour in good practice. But at the same time the findings of the initial assessments must not be regarded as inviolate. The term 'diagnostic therapy' has been increasingly used in recent years. Essentially this implies a degree of flexibility in determining the course of intervention (Howell and Dean, 1987). It necessitates an awareness of the changing nature of the child's language and of the interactive effect of the environment on this. A previously silent child, now exercising newly acquired verbal skills may impose considerable change on the attitude of those near to him. Another factor which needs to be taken into account is our own changing view of the nature of language disorder for this too will influence our methods even during the course of treatment. Damico (1988) offers a descriptive case study in which with a great deal of unjustified self-criticism he recounts his failure to recognise specific aspects of the language disorder of a child referred to him in 1976. The child was treated and subsequently discharged after satisfactory progress, and who then reappeared 6 years later with severe unresolved deficits which had previously been overlooked. According to the state of knowledge at the time of original referral, Damico's intervention was probably appropriate. We are all subject to a revision of our strategies and techniques in the light of on-going findings from research.

To procure comparative data from which change can be measured

It is a prime requirement of good practice that the course of therapy which has been undertaken should be monitored and evaluated. This is important both for anticipatory and retrospective reasons; in anticipation so as to determine the steps which should be taken in the future as a result of evaluation, and retrospectively in order to match the outcome against the content of past therapy. In Chapter 3, we have drawn attention to the special nature of monitoring, particularly with reference to ways in which it exceeds the role of re-evaluation.

An additional reason for this is the fact that a child may be subject to a change of therapist. To ensure continuity it is essential that the incoming therapist should have access to complete information regarding assessment and progress in order to minimise possible adverse effects of change. Issues of accountability which have been touched upon in Chapter 3 also enter into the need for data which measure progress. These are considered more fully at the end of this chapter.

For purposes of research

Knowledge about language disorders derived from research studies is still relatively sparse, especially when compared with scientific work emanating from professions of longer standing such as psychology or medicine. Happily there is a perceptible change now taking place with an increase in publication of valuable research from within the ranks of speech therapists. There is, however, an obligation to record meticulously our findings, strategies of intervention and outcome. This practice enables other workers to benefit and thus enhance the fruitfulness of their own work. Precepts which have been inculcated during undergraduate days should not be abandoned in practice on the pretext of pressure of work. The time-consuming factor is well recognised but for justification that this time is well spent the reader should refer to Crystal (1982a).

Methods of assessment

The preliminary interview

This is of course an important precursor of the form of assessment which may follow. It is not proposed in this text to enter into detailed discussion of interview techniques and procedures. The assumption is made that advanced students will already be familiar with these and that clinicians will in any case be employing them regularly. Guidance can be found in Hubbell (1981, Chapter 7), Darley and Spriestersbach (1978), Miller (1981) and in Warner, Byers Brown and McCartney (1984). Additional points which it may be useful to bear in mind are:

- It will not necessarily be the mother who provides biographical information about the child. Quite apart from those cases where the child for one reason or another is not living with the natural parents, changing cultural patterns coupled with high levels of unemployment may mean that the therapist's first line of contact will be with the father or with the cohabitee of the mother.
- It is also very possible that the child may come from a home where English is not the mother language and this could present problems for interviewing. There is considerable variation in pragmatic behaviours between differing cultures and a mismatch between the intention of the speaker and the code of the listener can give rise to misunderstanding.
- It is very likely that referral for speech therapy represents one link in a chain of previous referrals. There is therefore a need to establish, in advance if possible, what these other links are and to ascertain what information was obtained then. Because of the nature of language disorders, the therapist is probably functioning as a member of a team; it is therefore befitting to behave as such.

The interview is not a once-and-for-all occasion. Present practice favours active participation of parents in remediation and this should afford ample opportunity in the ongoing situation to obtain further information or to confirm or revise that previously given.

Descriptive language data

The following section deals specifically with assessment of language. It would, however, be wrong to regard this as a discrete entity. Language represents one very important aspect of behaviour which must be seen in relation to cognitive, emotional and social factors. Some aspects of these will have been deduced by the therapist in initial encounters with the child and from observation with the caregiver. Some characteristics of children who have impaired language are described in Chapter 1. There are two broadly defined methods commonly in use whereby detailed information about children's language may be obtained. These fall under the headings of:

1. Formal language testing.
2. Observational procedures (spontaneous language sampling).

Table 6.1 shows examples of some specific methods which can be placed under each heading.

Table 6.1 Examples of norm-referenced and naturalistic assessments

Norm-referenced tests	Naturalistic assessments
Auditory discriminatory test (Wepman, 1958)	Bloom and Lahey (1978)
ITPA (Kirk, McCarthy and Kirk, 1968)	Lund and Duchan (1983–87)
TROG (Bishop, 1983)	Muma Assessment Programme (Muma, 1979)
Boehm Test of Basic Concepts (1969)	
CELI (Carrow, 1974)	Miller (1981)
EAT (Anthony et al., 1971)	
RDLS (Revised, 1985)	

Contrary to some expressed beliefs, these two methods are not mutually exclusive. It is unfortunate that this view should prevail for the best outcome is that where each method stands in complementary relationship to the other. Each has its limitations and even if taken in conjunction they may not produce a definitive index of a particular pattern of language disorder. But they do serve as valuable pointers to the direction of remediation even though in the light of on-going treatment and growth in depth of knowledge of the child's language system, initial impressions may be modified.

Formal tests

These can be divided into:

● Norm-referenced tests.
● Developmental tests.
● Criterion-referenced tests.

During the early and mid-1960s there was a marked increase in the number and type of standardised language tests. For example, two which were in common use are the Illinois Test of Psycholinguistic Abilities (ITPA, Kirk, Macarthy and Kirk, 1968) and the Reynell Developmental Language Scales (RDLS, Reynell, 1977).

Almost invariably, these are normative referenced tests, that is to say, they compare an individual's performance with that of a number of other children matched for age and given the same tasks. Results of these tests are reported in standard scores and the number of standard deviations from the mean can then be computed. Alternatively the score can be expressed in percentiles. Some tests also include provision for a language age [e.g. RDLS and Test for Auditory Comprehension of Language (TACL) – Carrow (1973)]. Other tests rely on reported information, the data being obtained usually by questionnaire. The Vineland Maturity Scale (Doll, 1965) and the Verbal Language Development Scale (Mecham, 1968) are examples. Here the results are compared with age-related norms.

Such tests have value in identifying the existence of a problem as a first-line method following referral. It is possible that the child will already have had some type of screening test prior to this. The purpose of this will have been to determine whether referral to a speech therapist is an appropriate course of action. Reference has been made in Chapter 3 to the advantages and limitations of screening methods. It was pointed out that the multi-district study of Edwards *et al.* (1984) revealed only about 10% of inappropriate referrals. These findings were based on results of two standardised tests which were given at the initial assessment. Scores obtained on the Edinburgh Articulation Test (EAT, Anthony *et al.*, 1971) and on the TACL were tabulated against referring agents. A score of at least −1 standard deviation on either or both of these was taken to indicate a need for further investigation. On this basis, only 10.9% were found not to require further assessment. These 10.9% may have included children whose difficulties were not revealed by the tests, e.g. a disorder confined to syntactic level only, although this is unlikely. It might also be argued that the results showed selection bias in that therapists would hesitate to refer children in whom they did not observe deficits. There is also the possibility that children whose language problems were of a subtle nature were overlooked. Nevertheless, this low figure of 'no problem' does give confidence that, whatever screening methods are in current use by referring agents, they are reasonably effective.

Formal tests if well designed will offer categorical evidence of deficit, but will be unlikely to elucidate its precise nature. Also, because of their formality of design they cannot give a true indication of a child's communicative ability. Reliance on standard scores may also give a false picture of actual progress. This was apparent in the above-mentioned research study and was well exemplified by the case of a boy whose standard score at first assessment on the EAT was 67. Eighteen months later it was actually lower at 62. The qualitative analysis, however, showed a significant move towards more mature realisations. At the first assessment he produced 30 atypical (i.e. deviant and non-attributable to maturational lag) sounds. Eighteen months later this figure was reduced to 11. Similarly in the 'very immature' category, the initial figure of 16 was reduced to 12. 'Immature sounds', a less severe category, had however increased from 4 to 14 and there were now 2 'almost mature' realisations. The pattern therefore was one of progression towards an adult system, but none of these changes could be reflected in the total score since this only recognises adult realisations.

A frequently cited fact in favour of standard tests is that of objectivity, but as Muma (1978) observes, objectivity may be at the expense of relevance. However impeccable they may be in terms of validity and reliability, they do impose upon the child an artificial context in which he is required to demonstrate his understanding and/or use of language. Such artificiality applies not only to the content of the test but also to the setting in which it is given and this may have an indirect effect on results (Leonard *et al.*, 1978). Neither is a one-off test likely to produce a true picture of the child's communicative ability. Byers Brown (1985) observed that

> Screening for communication problems in infants is not a simple matter of counting response, but rather of putting together a number of observations, collecting evidence along a spectrum and not coming to a decision upon one pass/fail criterion. (p. 10)

Interaction of linguistic levels

Damico (1988) attributes his failure to recognise the true nature of his patient's language disorder in part to the tradition whereby language tests fragment levels into discrete components without recognition of the strong evidence against the autonomy of linguistic levels.

Crystal (1987) writes compellingly of the need to pay attention to the interaction of the different levels as well as to what is taking place at each level. Drawing on reports from a number of studies, he goes on to describe some of the possible interactions which can take place, for example, syntax/semantics/pragmatics; syntax/non-segmental/segmental phonology. Recent work has attempted to delineate subgroups of language reflecting this interaction and these were the basis of discussion in Chapter 5. Earlier, Panagos, Quine and Klich (1979) proposed a model in which interactive aspects of phonology and syntax were demonstrated in some language-disordered children.

Formal tests are unable to demonstrate these aspects; it is only through descriptive methods that they can be effectively charted.

Developmental tests

Tests which rely on developmental milestones have long been shown to have low validity (Weiner and Hoock, 1973). This reliance is based on the fallacy that children develop in a uniform linear fashion acquiring certain skills within given temporal parameters. Similarly, tests which relate to a posited language age are not really very helpful. In terms of design they are weak. One reason for this may be because at the lower age limit there are customarily more items than at upper limits. This of course reflects the more rapid changes which occur during early language development. Therefore a 1-year delay at chronological age 4;0 years may be the result of failure on as many as 12 items, whereas a 1-year delay at age 10;0 years may involve failure on only one or two items (McCauley and Swisher, 1984). Results are also misleading in that language age does not accurately mirror the child's language system. Take, for example, the case of a 5-year-old child who is stated to have a language age equivalence of 3 years. His language will not precisely replicate that of a normal 3 year old. In some respects it will be more advanced by virtue of his added life experience; in others it may be more retarded. Strategies which he may have developed along the line to cope with his deficit will also have an effect which is not age related on his language.

Strengths of formal tests

So, it might be asked, does a language test have any value? Provided that certain criteria are met it has a place in clinical assessment. First and foremost is the question of *selection*. Well-designed tests will have an accompanying manual describing in detail the population on which they have been standardised, the purpose for which they are intended and the sensitivity of the different subtests. Cultural differences may well influence performance and so this needs to be borne in mind. The user must also be quite clear as to the interpretation of the measurements used. After careful study we should be left with a clear indication of the appropriateness of the instrument for a particular individual. Familiarity with the contents of the manual is absolutely mandatory if credence is to be placed in quantifiable results.

Secondly, *instructions for administration* of the test must be followed rigorously. Therapeutic leanings are sometimes at variance with this precept, and knowledge of the child can lead towards securing an enhanced score. While this may be acceptable sometimes when employing naturalistic methods, objectivity is a strict criterion of formal testing. It is also important to remember that the resulting data give information about the child's language as it relates to *the model* on which the test is based. Another test designed on a different model may yield different results (see, for example, discussion in Bishop, 1986).

Summary

The use of norm-referenced tests will have the following advantages:

- As a first line measure to determine the extent although not necessarily the nature of the problem.
- To give an indication of the direction which subsequent more detailed investigation should take.
- To provide safeguards against variability in replication. This means that a child who has been tested on one occasion should be able to be retested with confidence by another user with the same test.
- To yield interpretable data for use in any estimates of accountability and effectiveness of therapy.
- They are usually quick and easy to administer.

Norm-referenced tests must nevertheless be regarded as adjuncts to other methods, for it is patterns of behaviour rather than levels of performance which determine how an individual functions linguistically (Muma, 1978).

Criterion-referenced tests

These differ from norm-referenced assessments in that comparative data are measured within the individual rather than against a hypothesised norm. Their purpose is to chart the changing language patterns of the child relative to certain predetermined tasks or goals (Bloom and Lahey, 1978). They are particularly valuable as reassessment measures during treatment in that they enable the clinician to estimate the stability of a specific linguistic behaviour which has been taught. Miller (1981) uses elicited imitation tasks for this purpose. Johnson and Schery (1976) have reported research on the development of grammatical morphemes in a group of language-disordered children. The most usual criteria set are frequently and proportion. In relation to production, Bloom (1973) set a frequency criterion of five or more multiword utterances representing a particular syntactic or semantic–syntactic relationship during a course of 5 hours' observation.

Until recently, criterion-referenced tests have not enjoyed the same degree of popularity as norm-referenced tests. This is because the latter are undoubtedly easier to administer, because specific directions as to procedures are laid down and raw scores can be obtained, converted into standard scores, percentiles or ranked. Criterion-referenced measures on the other hand demand a very solid basis of knowledge of the developing language system on the part of the assessor. In other words, there is a need to be very certain that the targets being set are appropriate. There is also a requirement for ingenuity in designing protocols through which it is possible to determine whether the target is being achieved. As a corollary to this goes the necessity of meticulous record keeping.

If, for example, the aim is to teach comprehension of prepositions, we might begin in a circumscribed manner with two contrasts, in/out – using objects as illustration and to provide context. When comprehension of this was stabilised in a particular situation, we might then move on to pictures and thence to wider contexts, proceeding from concrete to abstract situations.

Reference has been made to the use of relatively formal elicitation methods to establish structures, but there is some evidence that correct responses are not thereby generalised to free speech (Prutting, Gallagher and Mulac, 1975). Any reassessment needs to allow for this possibility. The above description indicates that criterion-referenced tests are very much interwoven into the fabric of therapy.

Turton (1983) states that one of the criticisms levelled against them is that because information is obtained in a naturalistic setting, they have neither reliability nor validity. He disputes this view on the grounds that repeated measures of a single behaviour serve to enhance rather than to diminish reliability, while the testing of such behaviour in depth confirms validity. Criterion-referenced testing does not carry with it a connotation of failure, such as is sometimes associated with norm-referenced tests in which the child is required to perform ever increasingly difficult tests until a ceiling of failure is reached (Haynes, 1986).

Spontaneous language samples

This is the starting point from which the majority of naturalistic assessments are derived. The notion of language sampling, although it has come into prominence in the last decade, is not in fact novel. McCarthy (1930) was one of the earliest workers to advocate this procedure. More recently, Bloom and Lahey (1978), Muma (1978), Miller (1981) and Lund and Duchan (1987) are among those who have developed and refined the methodology. Opinions vary as to what constitutes a representative sample both in terms of length and context. There is, however, general agreement that it should include more than one situation. Gallagher (1983), discussing contextual representativeness, considers that this needs to be determined individually for each child and that consequently a decision cannot be made until there has been an extensive preassessment to discover habits, interests etc. This she undertakes by means of a very lengthy questionnaire which is completed by the mother or caregiver.

Wells (1985), for his longitudinal Bristol study which was concerned with normally developing children, probably devised the ultimate method of obtaining as natural a sample as possible. For this, the study children were provided with a specially designed harness fitted with a radio microphone thereby giving them freedom of movement. This was worn during waking hours for a period of 24 hours before the observer visited the home. Thus almost every interchange between mother and child was picked up and relayed to a nearby receiver and then transmitted to a tape recorder. These recordings were subsequently transcribed by research linguists. Alas, such sophisticated resources are generally only available for large scale studies.

At a more realistic level a minimum of three situations seems to be generally recommended. Miller (1981) suggests

1. 15 minutes with the mother in free play.
2. 15 minutes with the clinician in free play.
3. 15 minutes with the clinician directing the child with questions and commands.

Presumably the last situation is for the purpose of eliciting specific features and/or estimating the level of verbal comprehension. The notion of providing specific contexts for each child is an attractive one, particularly as it leads easily into intervention. But for research purposes where a large number of subjects may need to be sampled, a more uniform situation is necessary. Most clinicians will have sets of toys which are developed and designed to appeal to both boys and girls. These were used in the study of Edwards et al. (1984); others may use pictures. The Bus Story (Renfrew, 1972) has proved to be an attractive way of obtaining preliminary information about both comprehension and production of connected speech.

Miller (1981) provides a wealth of ideas for situations likely to yield spontaneous language samples.

This type of descriptive assessment has many strengths and some limitations. Chief among the latter is the plea that it is a very time-consuming procedure. McCauley and Swisher (1984) report on a survey in which clinicians were asked about types of assessments used. While many were reported to favour a descriptive approach fewer than one-third actually used this form of analysis. The results of a questionnaire carried out in the UK by Baker (1988) yielded a similar response in relation to various types of language sample analyses: 87.9% of the respondents stated that they would ideally use this method at 6-monthly intervals, but in reality only about 33% of these did so. The time factor was the overriding reason advanced for this. A significant number stated that they would be helped greatly by computer-assisted analysis. The value of computers may, however, represent a somewhat enhanced view, for as those who are in the habit of analysing language samples well know, it is the transcription which is most onerous in terms of time and as yet there is no way of avoiding this manual task. This last study suffered from a very poor overall return, so the results may not be representative. They are likely to be biased in favour of language sampling, since the therapists attempting this type of assessment would be the most motivated to reply. Much of course depends on where priorities are placed in clinicial management. If clinicians bow to pressures of producing figures for statistical returns as a prime requirement, they are in danger of perpetuating a purely technical skills approach to their work. Intervention surely entails more than that. There is therefore an obligation to dispel the belief that language disorders can be treated in a prescriptive manner. That may mean a reduction in overall numbers, but an improvement in the quality of treatment.

Clinicians who adopt a combined approach of formal and descriptive assessment testify to the bettering of subsequent treatment and results. One of the strengths of naturalistic methods is that they allow for a holistic appraisal of the child's communicative behaviour. Reference has already been made to the interrelationship of language levels and to the necessity for assessment measures to take these into account. Muma (1983) maintains that descriptive assessment helps to focus on the individual nature of the child's disability. If an apparent phonological deficit is considered, for example, a sample of spontaneous utterance will provide far more information about a child's language system than will one derived from a set of stimulus words however representative they may be. Taken in isolation they will be unable to provide information about features such as co-articulation, relationship to morphology, or to syntactic complexity. For these reasons we would therefore wish to advocate the combination of both formal and informal methods in any assessment procedure.

Obtaining and interpreting the data

We have described methods by which samples of children's language may be obtained and have discussed the strengths and limitations of different procedures. But this represents only an intermediate stage in the process. A framework in which the data can be placed so as to give positive indications for remediation needs to be formulated. In other words what steps need to be taken in order to make sense from the information obtained?

There are several ways in which an analysis can be undertaken; formal testing, as has been pointed out, is one. Because many of the current tests of this nature have been comprehensively reviewed elsewhere, it is not proposed to consider them in detail here. Readers wishing to study such reviews should turn, for example, to Miller (1978.), Grunwell (1980b), Müller, Munro and Code (1981), McLaughlin and Gullo (1984).

Profiles

Profiles of children's language have become increasingly popular over recent years. *Chambers Thesaurus* in its 1987 edition gives the following among alternatives for the word 'profile': 'analysis–chart–contour–shape'. In terms of language any of these labels serves well as a description of the data obtained.

Profiling has the advantage that it can accommodate many aspects of language: cognitive, linguistic and biological. Within linguistic levels there are methods for profiling pragmatic features (Prutting and Kirchner, 1983) (though the protocol they describe is perhaps more of an inventory), semantic and syntactic (Miller, 1981). However, the profiles with which British speech therapists are likely to be most familiar are those devised by Crystal and his colleagues. There are four of these: PRISM which is concerned with semantics, LARSP, with syntax, PROPH, phonology and PROP which profiles prosodic features. In the 1982 edition of *Profiling Linguistic Disability*, Crystal has an introductory chapter in which he discusses the functions of profiles. They have two principal aims: the first is to identify the (linguistic) level of the child in relation to the level which should be achieved, and the second is to suggest a remedial path. The author emphasises the fact that these profiles do not specify in any way how remedial goals should be devised. In this respect they differ from language programmes which are much more prescriptive in nature and which tend to lack the flexibility necessary if each case is to be treated on an individual basis. Crystal sees the development of profiles as a 'compromise between clinical practice and academic diagnostic research', an attempt to bridge what appears at present to be a rather wide gulf.

Certainly the flexibility of profiling would appear to be one of its strengths, for it allows for investigation at a series of different levels of detail: what has been termed both molar and molecular analysis. From the first broad transcription, areas of particular difficulty can be pinpointed and these in turn can then be further investigated. At this stage, profiling systems which are adequate to assess all the processes described in Chapter 4 have not yet been developed. There is, for example no effective way in which the components of verbal comprehension can be profiled and therefore, pending outcome of research in this highly complex field, reliance is still placed upon tests. One possible framework within which the components of developmental language disorders can be assessed is shown in Table 6.2.

Table 6.2 Components of language assessment

Comprehension	↔	Integration	↔	Production
Attention		Perception		Pragmatics Intention to speak
Audition		Episodic memory		Linguistic planning
Vision		Long-term memory (Semantic)		Lexical Grammatical –
Proprioception				phonological
		Concept formation		Motor planning: articulatory

Pragmatics

An awareness of the importance of this aspect of communication has been slow to emerge. Since interest was aroused, however, we have been treated to a flood of differing theories, classifications and plans for assessment, leading, as McTear (1985) observes, to a state of considerable confusion.

Prutting (1982, cited in Prutting and Kirchner, 1983) developed a protocol which covers four broad areas of pragmatics. These are:

1. The utterance act: this relates to the way in which the act is presented, for example, the degree of fluency, voice quality, body language etc.
2. The propositional act which includes the linguistic aspects of the utterance, lexical choice, word order, contrastive stress.
3. The illocutionary act which conveys the speaker's intention.
4. The perlocutionary act which describes the effect of the act upon the listener.

Under these broad headings Prutting details examples which can be entered into the protocol (Prutting and Kirchner, 1983).

This protocol is directed mainly for use with older children, but it does include some discussion of its application both to developmental stages and to children with language disorders.

Lund and Duchan (1983) also include a pragmatics assessment. Although the contextual element is implicit in any analysis of pragmatics, these authors lay great stress upon this aspect and their suggested protocol which is also arranged in four areas includes the following:

1. Situational context.
2. Intentional context.
3. Listener context.
4. Linguistic context.

Lund and Duchan provide detailed description of each of these headings with examples of behaviours which may be subsumed under them.

One of the earlier assessments of functional language which is specifically related to very young children and which includes non-verbal behaviour is that developed by Halliday (1975) based on the development of his son, Nigel. The functions listed are:

Instrumental, e.g. a generalised request for an object.
Regulatory, e.g. a general request for action.
Interactional, e.g. vocalisation at the appearance of a person.
Personal, e.g. comments on objects.
Heuristic, e.g. requests for information.
Imaginative, e.g. pretend play.

These functions were observed to emerge between the ages of 9 and 18 months.

None of these protocols includes procedures for eliciting behaviours. Lund and Duchan (1983) state that it will depend upon which aspect is the focus of interest. They do, however, advise that several samples taken under differing contextual situations will probably be necessary.

Dewart and Summers (1988) have devised a pragmatics profile which provides a descriptive and qualitative assessment of the child's functional communication. It is based on a structured interview with the parent or caregiver. Dewart and Summers state that the responses obtained can then be used as a basis for planning intervention.

Although this section has described the assessment of pragmatics as a separate element of communication, as has already been pointed out in Chapter 4 it is extremely doubtful whether in reality it can be considered as such. Its close relationship to semantics makes a separate delineation both difficult and to some extent inappropriate. Bloom and Lahey's (1978) intersecting circles of form, content and use emphasise this.

Comprehension

Comprehension subsumes all other aspects of language. It involves the reception of phonological, grammatical and semantic information through sensory channels and its central integration, comparison and storage with past linguistic experience.

Assessment of comprehension without reference to language production poses many problems and, in any case, the wisdom of such a strategy is debatable. If, as has been maintained throughout this text, language disorders are seen to be on a continuum of severity, then the imposition of an artificial dichotomy between receptive language on the one hand and production on the other, will hardly be conducive to effective remediation. Well-documented research has shown that those disorders where receptive problems predominate tend to include production deficits as well (Eisenson, 1972, 1985). Conversely where expressive problems are salient, it is comparatively rare not to find some degree of associated comprehension difficulty (Bishop, 1979; Duxbury, 1986). The exceptions may be cases diagnosed as dysarthrias or verbal dyspraxias.

Underlying comprehension are a number of processes and conditions which it is maintained are necessary for understanding of language.

Attention

Reynell (1969) considered that the development of fully integrated attention was an essential substructure of comprehension. This was measured on an observational developmental scale ranging from simple single channel through to fully integrated multimodal attention which it is claimed is achieved by around 5 years of age (Cooper, Moodley and Reynell, 1978). A more detailed discussion of current theories of attention has been provided in Chapter 4.

Auditory perception

Evidence regarding the precise role played by auditory perception is conflicting, mainly because of the inadequacy of the measures used for its assessment. Rees (1973) points out that, as many of the tests are language based, failure could equally as likely be due to vocabulary as to discrimination deficits. Cromer (1978) would regard an apparent failure in auditory perceptual tasks as probably arising from the child's inability to deal with the hierarchical nature of language. The main problem, therefore, is what is being assessed? Traditionally the components of auditory perception which are examined are:

● Auditory discrimination.
● Auditory sequencing.
● Auditory memory.

Auditory discrimination

Methods for the assessment of this aspect are probably the least satisfactory in the auditory perceptual domain. In part, this is because an obvious gap may be present between the child's ability to extract information from the incoming signal and his reconstruction of this. Berry (1980) discusses the problems inherent in the assessment of auditory perception, particularly with reference to the processes which underlie the discrimination of sustained on-going speech. These are likely to be different from those which are effective for discrimination of isolated sounds.

Most of the auditory discrimination tests currently in use are based on word recognition. The child is either required to differentiate between two 'minimal pair' words on a same/different basis (Wepman Auditory Discrimination Test) or to select the stimulus word from a choice of three or four others, some of which are also minimally paired (Renfrew Auditory Discrimination Test). Morgan-Barry (1988) has recently produced a Test of Auditory Discrimination and Attention. This requires the child to select the stimulus word presented by the therapist from a choice of two pictures. The somewhat worrying feature of all these tests is the strong element of chance that the child will hit upon the right response (50% in the case of the Wepman test).

Locke (1980) reviews currently prevailing methods of assessing auditory perception and suggests criteria which should be met to avoid the shortcomings which he regards as endemic in these.

In the case of discrimination between minimal pairs, for example, there is an assumption that if the child responds correctly it is because he has recognised a difference between two consonants. It may be equally true that his discrimination is the result of differentiating between the frequencies of the following vowels.

He observes that many such tests fail to observe context sensitivity, i.e. that phonemes should be placed in identical phonetic environments for both perception and production. For example, if a child realises /rabbit/ as /wabbit/ then he should be tested on his perception of this contrast not just on some other w/r distinction, e.g. wing/ring. In a discrimination task, it is pointed out that there is a requirement to compare a sound just heard and stored in short-term memory with that in lexical long-term memory storage. This latter represents a composite of the sound which has been perceived on many different occasions and produced by many different people. An attempt to overcome this is to ensure repeated opportunity for discrimination of each sound. Locke also points out a fact which is well recognised by clinicians, namely that error may be the result of other factors such as inattention or sheer boredom. We are all familiar with the glazed look which comes with the tedium of repetitive performance associated with some of these tasks and with what seems like chance responses of 'same' or 'different'.

The critique of existing methods is ued by Locke to draw up eight criteria which are considered to be essential for assessment of auditory discrimination. These are employed in an accompanying paper in which he describes the design of two tests. The first (type 1) requires the child to compare the adult surface form of the utterance with his own internal representation. An important difference between this and other methods is that the stimulus words are based on the child's own production. This is derived from a prior articulatory test. There is therefore no standard list of stimulus words. The task includes differentiation between the correct production, his own and a closely related control, e.g. /thumb/ /fum/ /sum/. The second (type 2) speech perception test is based on discrimination of one adult surface form from another. It follows the design of many of the tests first devised at the Haskins Laboratories; this is essentially an ABX task where A represents one syllable, B a different one and X is either A or B (e.g. /pa/ /ba/ /pa/ or /pa/ /ba/ /ba/). Whereas type 1 task required the child to compare an adult form with his own internal representation, this test is designed to determine whether at an early stage of language acquisition he is able to recognise differences in adult forms. As Locke states: 'the clinical challenge is to separate the child who cannot detect a difference between two sounds from the child who detects a difference but considers it linguistically unimportant' (p. 456). In the first case, perceptual training may be indicated; in the second, there may be a need for phonological reorganisation.

Auditory sequencing

There are two considerations which are of importance in assessment of temporal features. The first is the rate at which the child is able to process the incoming information and the second his ability to reproduce it in the correct order. Stark, Tallal and Mellits (1985) have reviewed experimental work, much of it their own, which considers the relationship between auditory temporal factors and receptive speech. Their view is that children with specific language disability have difficulty in processing rapid incoming information. When the acoustic transition was less than 40 ms duration language-impaired children failed to discriminate, but when the duration was increased to 80 ms they were successful. Tests of auditory sequencing such as the subtest in the ITPA recommend an interval between digits. But it is important to bear in mind that the time factor may be one cause of poor performance. This test requires the subject to repeat the sequence of digits. Referring back to the model of processing it is equally possible that failure may be the result of encoding problems and not of input.

Auditory memory

Limitations of auditory memory have also been cited as being contributory to effective comprehension of language. The most usual way of assessing this is to get the child to repeat sentences of increasing length. There are differences between assessment that requires repetition of isolated words or strings of digits and those which rely on sentence repetition. In the latter case, performance is likely to be better, for the child will be able to make use of semantic cues.

Whilst many researchers regard impaired auditory perception as one of the principal contributory features of severe language disorders, others would attribute the results of assessments such as these described above to other causes. Cromer (1978) would place them in a model of cognitive processing and would see the impairment as evidence of the child's inability to deal with the hierarchical nature of language. Such difficulties have also been construed as showing a lack of metalinguistic awareness (Van Kleek, 1984; Howell and McCartney, 1989).

Syntactic comprehension

The two assessments of grammar most widely in use currently are the Test for Reception of Grammar (TROG, Bishop, 1983) and the Test for Auditory Comprehension of Language (TACL-R, Carrow, 1985). Each covers a range of grammatical and morphological structures which the subject identifies from a selection of pictures in response to a spoken stimulus. The Action Picture Test (Renfrew, 1988) has long been popular as a screening test of grammar and content. It has recently been revised and restandardised by the author.

Wiig and Semel have written extensively on the assessment of language within a cognitive processing framework.

Language production

Turning to language production, not unexpectedly there is somewhat less confusion, for at least here observable behaviour is being described. Assessment methods have evolved from standardised tests (e.g. North Western Syntax Screening Test, Lee, 1969; Carrow Elicited Language Inventory, 1974; Edinburgh Articulation Test, Anthony et al., 1971), through to profiling procedures which are currently more favoured. Such profiles are derived from the transcription of language samples obtained from naturalistic observation or from elicited methods. With the increasing use of profiles, there has been a move away from equating results with specific language ages. Rather, they are interpreted as representing particular stages in language production. Crystal, Fletcher and Garman (1976) delineated seven such stages of syntactic development. The original version has been modified by 1982 in some respects (see note in Crystal, 1982b, for details). The interdependence of the levels of language production is implicit in the profiles developed by a number of workers. Bloom and Lahey (1978) emphasise this aspect within their interesting circles of content, form and use. Crystal (1987) has more recently acknowledged the importance of considering language in an interactive framework. It is interesting to note that, as late as 1981, he was adopting what he termed 'a fairly narrow view' (p. 97), namely, by treating levels discretely, although he does consider the possibility that this may not be the most fruitful way of describing disability. Later in the same text, he discusses the relationship between grammar and semantics and acknowledges the problems which are sometimes apparent in isolating each factor.

Miller (1981) discusses procedures for analysing speech samples. Among general analyses he includes mean length of utterance (MLU; Brown, 1973). For this, the mean number of words or morphemes is counted for each tone-group and the mean is computed for 100 such utterances. The resulting figure is then assigned to a stage which corresponds to a predicted developmental age. The measure is still frequently cited in research studies, but its reliability is open to question. Miller (1981) emphasises the need to guard against over-interpretation of the results and Brown himself has noted that interpretation is only reliable between levels of 1.01 and 4.49. He has also indicated that a complete revision of the levels is proposed. It is noteworthy that Miller advocates further analysis of the sample in terms of content and syntactic complexity before interpreting results. A number of factors may influence these. Length of utterance does not of itself tell us much about its structure and is therefore not particularly useful as a prelude to remediation. A very short MLU may arise for reasons other than linguistic deficit. For example, because of respiratory restrictions, a dysarthric child may well produce truncated tone-groups. In 1987, Miller noted that an MLU matching strategy, while focusing on developmental change, limits the way in which language disability may be described. He discussed the types of error in grammatical production and the possibility of delineating subtypes of language disorder. Fletcher and Garman (1986) using LARSP as a starting point are concentrating research on these aspects.

Lexical retrieval

German (1985, 1987) has carried out considerable research in this field. Her assessments were based on the protocol devised by Wiig and Semel (1980) (since modified). This relies on naming of geometric shapes, colours etc. and is intended for children aged 5;0–10;0 years. In any such test it is important to differentiate between recognition and retrieval. Failure may be the outcome of either of these processes.

Prosodic features

It is interesting to note that in the taxonomy of measurement he proposes, Miller includes many non-segmental features. All too often assessment procedures either overlook these or tack them on the end as a sort of afterthought, so that they then tend to receive only cursory attention. This does not make linguistic sense, for it is generally acknowledged that in the hierarchy of development, prosody precedes segmental phonology both in comprehension and production. Crystal (1982b) has devised a prosodic profile (PROP) which is valuable as an indicator for intervention. It requires the transcription into tone units of about 100 utterances. These are analysed on LARSP principles into clause, phrase and word types. The location of the nuclear tone (tonicity) and the pitch direction (tone) are noted. PROP is concerned mainly with intonational aspects of prosody. It is useful, however, to assess other features such as rate, pause and contrastive stress. This can be done on a qualitative basis. The importance of this is particularly apparent in the case of analysis of a phonological/ syntactic disorder. It must be emphasised that because there is so little research data available on the development of prosody, other than for intonation (e.g. Allen and Hawkins, 1978), it is not advisable to ascribe a developmental age to these tasks. Crystal (1987), referring to an MRC study which he undertook, reported that prosodic impairment proved to be the most significant discriminating feature in a group of 30 language-handicapped children.

Koike and Asp (1981) report an experimental test (Tennesse Test of Rhythms and Intonation Patterns, T-Trip) which requires children to listen to and imitate pre-recorded variations of rhythm and intonation using the syllable /ma/. Their initial report gives results for 10 children of age range 3;0–3;11 and for 10 aged 5;0–5;11. Not unexpectedly, the older children achieved higher scores.

Semantic features

If assessment of syntax presents problems because of an insubstantial theoretical base (Miller, 1987), these are even more apparent in the case of semantic assessment. At the present time, only tentative inroads have been made and as yet no truly working method of assessment is available. In part this is due to the inherent difficulties in analysing the constituents of 'meaning' which by tradition have such strong philosophical connotations. In his description of the underlying theory, Crystal (1981) cautions against the common confusion which exists between comprehension and semantics. A comprehension test is not a semantic analysis, though semantic features may form a part of it.

His profile (PRISM, 1982) is subdivided into two sections; PRISM-G comprises semantic–grammatical items while PRISM-L categorises semantic–lexical features. The latter covers 16 pages and is an attempt to provide an inventory of the possible range of lexical fields which might be covered by teachers and therapists with children. It is noted that in order to obtain a representative sample, elicitation tasks will need to be undertaken in addition to that obtained from spontaneous speech. A study of the theoretical basis and of the profiling technique, leaves the reader not a little daunted by the complexities of the analysis and in particular of the interpretation of some of the items in the lexical section. A computer analysis would help, but as has been mentioned in connection with other profiles, the time-consuming transcription would still have to be under-taken. Aldred (1983) carried out an interesting small study of intervention in which she used PRISM as part of her assessment procedure. Her group of six children of age range 3;1–4;10 years divided into those with predominantly expressive problems and those with receptive difficulties.

The 'expressive' group was characterised by a heavy reliance on clause structures, semantically high in content with a preponderance of information loaded lexemes: 'read books. Play train.' In contrast, the predominantly 'receptive' group revealed restricted semantic functions. There was a high proportion of spontaneous to responsive utterances, over-use of coordination, tag questions and stereotypes: 'home in there, it down and out.' Aldred concludes that, taken in conjunction with other assessments of pragmatics and structure, PRISM has good potential for delineating subgroups of language disorder.

Miller (1981) describes what appears in some respects as a parallel taxonomy for semantic analysis. This is based on De Villiers and De Villiers' (1978) definition of referential and relational meaning. The former defines the link between words and the objects they stand for and the latter concerns the network of relationships existing among concepts, words and sentences. As a measure of referential meaning, Miller suggests a type-token procedure, as, for example, that published by Templin in 1957. A framework for relational meaning is proposed by Rutherford, Schwartz and Chapman (cited in Miller, 1981). This lists 21 semantic categories or fields as compared with 61 in PRISM.

Assessment of early vocabulary

This is a procedure which has found favour with some researchers. It is certainly an easier method although the results lack the depth found in the semantic analyses described above. Locke (1975) includes a first-words assessment in her living language programme. This is a 100-word vocabulary list which includes nouns, verbs, prepositions and adjectives in that order. There is a wide variation among children who are developing language along normal lines and for this reason she sets a surprisingly low baseline of 10 words at 2;0 years. This scheme emphasises the use of vocabulary with less focus on how meaningful is its use. It will be interesting to refer to Price's findings in which she is investigating categories of error, using the Locke list as a starting point (Price, personal communication).

A limitation of vocabulary counts is that isolated words do not allow for contextual meaning. A situation familiar to most clinicians is that in which the child has been taught a vocabulary list by well intentioned parents. These are in effect labels with little regard to relational meaning.

Phonology

One of the most widely used phonological profiles in current use is that developed by Grunwell (Phonological Assessment of Child Speech, PACS, 1982a). This is based on a contrastive analysis of elicited speech with options for further different types of analysis. Potentially it offers a very detailed breakdown of a child's phonological system. This strength, however, may to some extent be self-defeating in that clinicians, as we have seen, tend to be put off by the complexity of such procedures. As students, unless they happen to be taught by the authors, they do not really have the opportunity to develop a realistic working familiarity with the methodology and therefore rarely feel confident enough to use them routinely. These comments apply to many of the procedures described above, but probably phonology lends itself more readily to an even greater degree of detail.

Other systems, equally time consuming, include a generative approach (Smith, 1973), and a naturalistic analysis based on Stampe's work which has been developed by Ingram (1981). Process analysis has been written up extensively by Shriberg and Kwiatkowski (1982) (see Grunwell, 1982b for review and critique) and Weiner (1979).

In commenting on the realities of undertaking such detailed assessments, it is not our intention to minimise in any way their value. On the contrary, they are very rewarding in that they provide a direct line to plans for remediation. Furthermore they add information which strengthens the evidence for delineation of subgroups. Grunwell has suggested parallels between phonological development and the stages of syntactic develop-ment proposed by Crystal, Fletcher and Garman. She rightly cautions, as indeed do others, against a too rigid regard for age norms.

A disadvantage of many phonological assessments is that they are based on single-word samples. Crystal's PROPH does allow for the analysis of connected speech though this is not obligatory. This system also includes analysis of vowels whereas many others concentrate on consonants on the grounds that vowels are so heavily influenced by dialect.

An example of the limitations of single word sampling was apparent in a case study described by Morgan-Barry (1988) in which data using the PACS stimulus words, and that obtained from spontaneous speech yielded differing patterns. Probably a sample of ongoing speech plus an elicited sample offers the most reliable evidence.

A composite scale which is designed to measure the expressive language of children aged between 15 months and 5;0 years is proposed for publication late in 1988. This is the Bristol Language Development Scales (Gutfreund, 1988). The assessment claims to measure pragmatics, seman-tics and syntax. It derives from the Bristol Language Development programme (Wells, 1985). Reference has been made at intervals through-out the chapter to metalinguistic aspects of language. At the present time, workers who adopt a metalinguistic approach rely for the most part on formal testing methods, for they maintain that these do tap the child's ability to reflect on his language. Van Kleek (1984) cites the Wepman Auditory Discrimination Test as offering the child opportunity to consider carefully the nature of the stimulus words before responding. Howell and

Dean have designed a remedial procedure (Metaphon) for phonological disorders (forthcoming 1990). Using natural process analysis they base their work on Piagetian constructs and on increasing the child's metalinguistic awareness of the sound system. It is mainly in the course of intervention that the metalinguistic strategies are encouraged.

Accountability

Our concern throughout this chapter has focused on the need to provide the optimum conditions and opportunity for the investigation of the child's behaviour so that appropriate remediation may follow as a natural corollary. It is also necessary to consider the issue of accountability particularly with reference to evaluation of such remediation for all clinicians have an obligation to ensure that to the best of their ability they are providing an appropriate service both to the children they treat and to the authorities that employ them (see Chapter 3).

In its narrowest sense, accountability requires an unwarranted measuring of work carried out. Siegel, Katsuki and Potechin (1985) observe that 'value questions meet us at every turn. Concern about which clients we should serve, what the criteria should be for accountability, how to measure the cost of services against the quality of life of clients'. This last factor is particularly relevant and is one which seems to be at variance with the less acceptable facets of accountability. That changes in human behaviour cannot be so easily numerically recorded is to state the obvious and language presents a particularly complex field of behaviour. Efficacy studies of acquired language disorder have yielded disappointing results in terms of quantifying the value of therapy, but enlightened discussion has cautioned against taking such figures at their face value. Weakness of design and a multiplicity of variables has confused the findings. Additionally, as we have sought to emphasise, communicative ability adds up to more than a set of language scores.

A broader definition of accountability is described by Douglass (1983). Legislative aspects are discussed, but he goes on to say that accountability requires a personal commitment on the part of the clinician to justify the quality of the service he or she offers to the person with a communication handicap.

Because of the differing pattern of health care within the USA as compared with the current (1988) system within the UK, namely the widespread range and use of private health insurance, the impression is given that North American colleagues are required to provide evidence of treatment efficacy more routinely, and that in order to do this, they have, albeit reluctantly, to rely very much on test results. Should speech therapy services ever suffer privatisation in the UK, and possibly also within a redesigned National Health Service it may come about that British speech therapists could face similar pressures.

Chapter 7
The Nature and Timing of Intervention

Summary

This chapter discusses the principles underlying intervention and discusses the advantages and limitations of the range of facilities that is presently available including language units, special schools and routine health service provision. Comparison is made between statutory rights of language-disordered children in the UK and the USA. The subtypes of language disorder described in Chapter 5 are further considered with reference to appropriate types of intervention.

The management of children with developmental language disorders is dependent for its success upon two overall factors:

1. The presence of well trained and skilled professionals in all the relevant disciplines.
2. Systems of health care and education that allow the expertise to be available to those who need it.

Within these broad provisions there are all sorts of special arrangements, techniques and tactics.

As has been indicated throughout this text, the academic study of language disorders occurs in all the developed countries and many of the same types of investigations are carried out and conclusions reached. The principles of intervention derived from these conclusions are also common to a number of different nations. Were it not so, the study of language disorders in developing children would have little validity since the conditions described could only be related to individual cases. Where we see differences, they are of application and emphasis. Nevertheless, the service provision is basic to the philosophies and attitudes of professionals involved since one generation creates it and subsequent generations are influenced by it. With regard to colleagues within the European

Community, this commonality is particularly important for, by 1992, it is likely that there will be some form of general recognition of professional qualifications in speech pathology across all member states. Already there are preparations for this and in order to ensure a sharing of experience the British College of Speech Therapists has participated in a number of meetings with European colleagues. Some university departments have also collaborated in an annual teaching programme where speech pathologists from a number of European countries have taken part. There is the intention that such a scheme should lead to shared qualifications at a postgraduate level.

While emphasising shared experience, within systems of health care among developed nations, however, we find considerable differences, although there is an overall trend towards early identification of and treatment for all developmental disabilities. Within the field of education there is also a common leaning which is having important consequences for those with language disorders. This is the integration of handicapped children into regular schools.

The philosophy of integration is unexceptionable since it aims to allow all children to participate fully in the life of the community and not to suffer isolation or stigma through disability. The practice can, however, be very penalising to those very children it purports to help. Integration of the handicapped depends for its success on excellent support services. These kinds of services are extremely vulnerable to economic cuts. We must view with alarm, therefore, any attempt to integrate children with special needs into regular schools at a time when the education system is starved of money and resources. Our language-disordered children are particularly vulnerable because we have not yet developed enough good techniques of remediation to propagate them with assurance. We still need time to examine how language-disordered children respond to specific management strategies and this cannot be done if the children are struggling to survive.

At the time of writing, England is also struggling with the development of a national curriculum. There is concern as to the extent to which this prevailing wind will be tempered to the shorn lamb. Since children with language disorders lack the ability to integrate their language skills and place them at the benefit of further learning, they may forever be running into particular problems of comprehension and execution. Not all their skills will be retarded to the same degree, but the extent to which learning is affected cannot always be anticipated. The need of those with language disorders is for flexible provision which can cover structured language teaching as well as other educational measures. Flexibility is also needed in the timing of educational procedures and this is where the national curriculum presents some problems.

We must therefore continue to propagate the need for special language units where children can be given intensive help and where techniques of therapy and teaching can be developed and tested. It will probably always be necessary to retain a few residential special schools for those children whose problems are so profound that they need protection from the demands of the normal community until they have developed some learning strategies together with sufficient insight and maturity for survival. Protected communities are also necessary for children with severe medical problems or conditions which require a particular combination of medical, educational and social surveillance. Our existing facilities include individual therapy, remedial teaching, language unit placement and placement within a special school for children with disorders of communication. These facilities operate on the assumption that children who have failed to develop language in the normal way can be taught the sequence of abilities which should have developed spontaneously. They also operate upon the assumption that children can be trained to compensate for impaired language skills in a better way than they can evolve for themselves. A further assumption is that language-disordered children are penalised by society and so society owes them some special care in exchange. We do not propose to challenge this third assumption but the first two will be discussed.

Can language be taught?

This is a question posed by Harris (1984) in an essay which goes right to the heart of the matter. Harris argues that teaching and traditional forms of language intervention are incompatible with the development of natural language abilities in language-disordered children. Thus interventionalists should concentrate upon facilitating development and 'then document the emergence of each child's personal language curriculum' (p. 249). If we are to stimulate language along normal lines, our success must depend on the extent to which we can stimulate the children to behave like normal language users. Unless the child can take over the language learning in a very active way, we can do little more than give a set of linguistic structures and as much communicative success as we can muster. Some children are going to be able to contribute more actively to language learning than others not just by virtue of temperament and intelligence but because of the nature of the underlying disorder. The more impaired are those areas underlying comprehension, semantic and pragmatic skills, the more likely is the child to be perpetually restricted in language since he is not able to make language discoveries. We have to accept that there are only some aspects of language which can be explicitly taught whether by capitalising on the skills of the mother or by later involving the child in a scientifically based and explicitly principled teaching programme. Language is characterised by structure and creativity. The basic rules have to be mastered in order that it can become the tool for communication, the expression of thought and all sorts of imaginative enterprises. The child needs to know his language and be able to reflect upon it. Normally developing children, having mastered the basic language structures and processes, will use them in all sorts of communal as well as individual activities. The pursuit of these activities will stimulate more variety of language forms. For example, young children coming together in pretend play will use politeness forms and verbal reasoning requiring a higher level of performance than is encountered among other exchanges (Garvey and Kramer, 1988). They are constantly stretching themselves cognitively and linguistically in the attempt to achieve together those goals which would be impossible apart. Their language development is not being stimulated by goals set by other people but by their own needs and interests.

Language teachers and therapists have recognised that natural situations, or those situations which occur naturally during the development of normal children, are necessary to stimulate normal language growth. This is very evident in the shift of remedial approaches from the modification of behaviour to the promotion of interaction. It is not useful to attempt to graft language structures or even language strategies on to an organism that is not receptive to new experiences. The difficulty was first perceived as one of generalisation. Individual components of language could be taught, but the difficulty lay in getting the child to make use of these components in his normal behaviour and to integrate them into a developing language system. The feasibility of helping language development through specified periods of intervention in a clinical setting has been severely questioned. Speech therapists are particularly vulnerable to such criticism since this is the way so many of them work. We may wonder, however, whether the individual clinician, working interactively with a young child in the presence of his mother, is more or less likely to achieve some gains in language growth than is the person who administers a specific teaching programme to a group of children in a class, even if it is administered every day. On the evidence of changes in test scores after a period of 18 months, the study of Edwards *et al.* (1984) found no significant difference in progress between group (intensive language class) therapy and individual treatment. These results, however, are qualified by (1) small numbers and (2) no control over the type of therapy given in these settings. It can be said, however, that it is unlikely to be the setting which dictates the effectiveness of the language therapy, but the extent to which this therapy can stimulate language learning in the child. Each facility may have a use. What is needed are good selection criteria or very good reasons for a child being given a particular type of intervention by a particular person in a particular place.

Effective intervention

Reviews of intervention approaches and discussions as to their success emphasise the importance of selecting the approach which is most appropriate for the individual case. Leonard (1981), writing about a number of approaches then current, found several to be effective when used appropriately, suggesting that their value was relative rather than absolute. Effective intervention resulted in language gains and had cumulative learning effects. Intervention approaches included:

- Imitation based approaches.
- Expansion approaches.
- Focused stimulation approaches.
- General stimulation approaches.

Fey, in a text written 5 years later (Fey, 1986), discusses the whole process of language intervention, citing different approaches used in the accomplishment of different goals. For example, in training content—form interactions, there are trainer-oriented approaches, child-oriented approaches and hybrid approaches. If the goal is to facilitate responsiveness to a conversation partner there are operant approaches, a number of which Fey specifies and child-oriented approaches as previously described by the author. Fey sees intervention as employing a range of procedures. These procedures are brought into being by an agent (clinician, teacher, parent) who 'stimulates or responds to a child in a manner that is consciously designed to facilitate development in areas of communication ability that are viewed as being at risk of impairment' (p. 49). Fey, in using this definition, accepts that a variety of approaches will be used by clinicians operating under markedly different conditions and with differing theoretical orientations. Since there is such a number of alternatives among intervention procedures, it is not easy to select the right one in every case. Perhaps it is even more important to avoid the wrong one. Kirk, writing about written language in 1983, makes a point that is also applicable to spoken language. If instruction is faulty, it may actively impede the learning of children whose preparatory skills are inadequate or barely adequate. To use a very simple illustration, if we choose a delayed speaker aged 3 years or so, who is just starting to use words referentially and try to take him through babbling procedures to improve his motor control, we are likely to affect his language learning adversely. On the other hand, if we continue to encourage points and grunts with no attempt at articulatory shaping, we are not helping the child to achieve conventional utterances. Intervention is therefore all about decisions. We are particularly aware of this with the younger children because of the possibility of doing harm through not appreciating the nature of the emerging problem. While it is possible to do harm at any age, we have less excuse when the child is older with more signs to offer us as to his needs.

When we select children for intervention, we must believe that our timing is right as well as our procedures appropriate. This applies at a number of different stages. The first decision is whether to intervene or to wait. The next may be to decide how intensively to intervene. If the child is very young, should our procedures be home based or centre based? If the child is older, should he attend a clinic or a unit or class for the language disturbed? Unfortunately, some of these questions remain academic because there may be so few treatment possibilities open to the child. This concentrates decisions about selection. Which children should receive the benefit of our sparse resources?

Admission criteria

All special schools catering for children with primary or specific disorders of language have fairly stringent criteria for admission. Here are the criteria for entry to a non-maintained residential school (Lea, 1986):

- Intelligence is at least within the average range (assessment does of course take account of children's verbal comprehension difficulties).
- Hearing thresholds are above 40 dB on the speech-related frequencies.
- There is no primary emotional disturbance or behavioural disorder.
- There is no primary stammer.
- There is no evidence of autism.
- Children are physically able to attend to their own needs and to join in the normal day-to-day activities of the school.

Aims

The school aims to deal intensively with the children's problems so that most transfer to mainstream education before school-leaving age. Similar criteria operate in a school that comes under the aegis of a local education authority. Here the children are resident for 5 days of the week and arrangements are being made for part-time attendance where this is practicable. Children with receptive and expressive disorders are eligible, but should be free from hearing impairment, severe generalised learning difficulties, childhood psychosis or autism, severe emotional disturbance or physical handicap. The school prospectus recognises that children with these conditions are likely to have severe language-learning difficulty, but very reasonably points out that it would be impossible for a small school to provide appropriate teaching and therapy for such a range of handicapping conditions. Such restrictions are common to special schools of this nature, not only in the UK but also in the USA and in Australia. Ellis Robinson representing Australia gave a similar list when discussing the Australian provision in 1987.

Curricula for special schools and language units

The more closely the school pursues the aim of eventual integration of the children into mainstream schooling, the more closely must it adhere to the mainstream curriculum. It must therefore attempt to combine a wide and varied curriculum with specialised language teaching. The residential special schools may concentrate on a more specialised aspect with use of augmentative communication systems. Individual therapy is prescribed as well as the participation of the speech therapist in the language activities of the classroom. Although integration back into the regular school community is the aim of the special school, there are a number of other goals. These are set out in one school prospectus (Ewing School, Manchester, 1988) as follows:

● To develop in our pupils as full an understanding and use of language as possible. To give them confidence to use what language they have in the widest possible social context. For a few very handicapped, this may mean encouraging skills in compensating for spoken language which may always be a difficult medium for them.
● To develop as far as possible the basic skills of reading, writing and number. Again for a few pupils this may well mean concentrated effort in learning what is absolutely essential for them for life beyond school.
● Inclusive of the first two points, the wider curriculum is aimed at helping pupils who remain through to school-leaving age to lead interesting and useful lives as members of the community; also to encourage the development of personal interests and advanced skills to the highest possible level of competence.

It was pointed out in our first chapter that those who encounter language-disordered children for the first time in a special school setting may receive a much more positive impression than they would if they were seeing individual children experiencing failure in the normal school. All special schools want to receive their pupils before they experience too much demoralisation through failure. Lea (1986), writing to this point, refers to the growing reluctance of some authorities to continue sending severely language-disordered children to residential special schools. This could be coincidental upon the mainstreaming philosophy and the lack of money for education and must therefore be viewed with suspicion. Lea does state, however, that if residential special schools are to compaign for candidates it is incumbent on them to keep abreast of modern thought, practice and technology and to develop and share expertise.

The move away from residential provision could be seen as a positive one if it meant that all local authorities were committed to setting up sufficient and appropriate language units within their schools. This is hardly the case, although provision is certainly improving and likely to continue.

Language units

The charitable organisations ICAN (Invalid Children's Aid Nationwide) and AFASIC (Association For All Speech Impaired Children) have recently issued guidelines for language units. ICAN's guidelines follow a survey carried out in 1987 (Hutt and Donlan) into provision. The guidelines ask a number of important questions which must be satisfactorily answered before a language unit should be established. They relate to type of handicap, availability of classroom and other space, involvement of head teacher and other staff of the school in which the unit is to be placed, availability of suitably qualified teaching staff or provision for training them, availability of a suitably qualified educational psychologist to be involved in admission and discharge procedures and also in general support. This preliminary thinking is related to the lack of overall direction in the setting up of language units, with each local authority having its own standards and determining its own criteria for the selection of both children and staff. The situation is exacerbated when the language unit is a joint venture between LEA and District Health Authority. Lack of uniformity is also a point made in the AFASIC guidelines which indicate, however, that local authorities are now seeking help in the setting up of language units and require examples of good practice. With the combined proselytising activities of AFASIC and ICAN in combination with other organisations like VOCAL, which has funded research into needs, we may hope to see a more clearly defined and cohesive policy towards language unit provision. All recommendations suggest that language units should be attached to mainstream schools with provision for gradual integration and with opportunities to share as many activities as are feasible. Provision is recommended for children upwards of 3 years with priority being given to the age range 3;0–7;0 years by authorities establishing units for the first time. Once criteria for infant and junior level provision are established, units should be set up in the middle school.

The ICAN guidelines recognise that many children with below average non-verbal ability also have specific language disorders. They therefore suggest that units for these children be established in schools for children with moderate learning difficulties.

The guidelines recognise that language impairment will be present in some degree where there is:

● Physical disability.
● Severe or moderate learning difficulty.
● Behavioural and/or other emotional problems.

● Hearing loss.
● Autism.
● Severe reading and spelling difficulty sometimes known as dyslexia.
● Other handicaps less frequently.

It is assumed that children suffering from these difficulties are allocated provision on the basis of their primary disability. Also excluded from language unit provision should be those children who are learning English as a second language and who do not have a primary language disorder.

These exclusions are in accord with the residential school directive and, in theory at least, are sound. Naturally where children with other handicaps are being severely penalised by language impairment, the position is more difficult to justify. Schools and units which exist specifically for the language disordered must nevertheless use stringent criteria or they will end up helping no one and providing nothing. It is to be hoped that techniques developed therein may be applied fruitfully to other populations of language-impaired children.

ICAN then suggests another group which should be excluded and this leads to rather more problems. This is the comparatively large group of children with language delay arising from 'minimum of linguistic demands being made during preschool years'. In order for this criterion to be applied justly, the succeeding recommendations need to be followed very closely. These are: that the child be placed in a mainstream school which supplies a basic curriculum and, within this, that there should be extra group teaching from a support teacher. Identification should be made of areas which need enrichment and suitable experience and materials provided. The speech therapist should be available, either as a consultant or to give individual therapy as required. Such children would be well catered for in the Birmingham scheme (Locke, 1989) as described in Chapter 3. Where no such facilities exist for regular teacher/therapist consultation, these children will fare very poorly. Nevertheless the recommendation is correct. Children who are capable of learning language through general stimulation should not be placed in classes where the emphasis is upon compensatory strategies.

Finally, it is recommended that children with severe articulation problems arising from dysarthria alone should only be placed in language units if no alternative is available. The prognosis for these children is usually poor and so their long-term sojourn in a language unit could deprive children of the means whereby they could learn to master the language system and thus function effectively in mainstream school. While the ruling is not questioned the terminology here is rather confused. Dysarthria is not solely an articulatory problem; indeed this may be secondary to other deficits of respiration and phonation. Language disorder is also a very likely concomitant. It seems likely too that, if there is such a severe neurogenic language disorder, there will be some degree of associated physical handicap which would place such a child within the aegis of a school for physically handicapped children and where it is hoped he would receive appropriate teaching and speech therapy.

These considerations bring up the whole question of prognosis, which has a place in decision making, though exactly what that place is, is by no means clear. There are a number of children whose language disorders suggest a poor prognosis but who are entitled to help. We are not ready to exclude children from language therapy or teaching because of possible poor prognosis and it is to be hoped we never will be. Prognosis may reasonably affect the nature and aims of therapy and the site of delivery. Schery (1985) makes the point that remedial programmes should be modified to meet the needs of children who are not likely to make good progress. However, the list of predictive factors which Schery gives have not been widely agreed. They were the result of a large statistical study of language correlates which has been challenged on a number of grounds (Kahmi, 1985; Bishop, 1987a).

Paul and Cohen (1987) reviewed a group of children with serious language disorders who had received full initial evaluations at an average age of 6;5 years. The average age of the 18 children seen at follow-up was 14;2 years. The subjects had originally been placed in two groups. One group consisted of children with developmental language disorders, but no social deficits. The other group was deemed atypical developmental language disorder since the children showed social withdrawal, poor or fleeting social relations and some of the sensory and motor responses of autism. All subjects had previously been diagnosed as 'aphasic'. Paul and Cohen do not discuss their atypical group in relation to semantic–pragmatic language deficits. However, they do state that none of the children satisfied the full criteria for infantile autism. It is possible, however, that they resembled severe cases of semantic–pragmatic disorder.

These authors found that the children with developmental language disorder and a high non-verbal IQ had a better outcome than those with low non-verbal IQ in terms of language growth and educational function. They also state that receptive skill together with intellectual capacity seem to be more important determinants of school placement than is speech since children with good understanding can function in less restrictive settings even when their expressive skills are less advanced: 86% of the low IQ developmental disordered language group and all of the atypical group had found placement in highly restrictive special day or residential schools. Only 50% of the high IQ children with developmental language disorders had been placed outside regular schools. The IQ appeared to account for a great deal of the differences among the groups. The low IQ children differed from the atypical group only in degree of communicative intent. The latter group remained seriously deficient in communication. Paul and Cohen therefore argue that deficiency in early social skills has prognostic value in relation to communication. However, since both the low IQ groups showed poor language outcome, social skills do not emerge as a strong predictor of language growth.

This study has obvious implications for those concerned with provision. Its findings lend support to the ICAN recommendation for language units to be set up in schools for slow learning children. When educational authorities find that they have to choose between setting up units for one group or another, the implications are less clear. One argument suggests that children with good language prognosis should have the advantage of the best facilities available since they can benefit most and make a speedier return to mainstream school. Another argument is to give the most comprehensive and intensive help to children who may do poorly because they would not survive in any other situation. A very cogent point to make is that all members of staff working in schools or units where a comparatively small number of children are receiving intensive remediation, need to see progress. If only those children with a poor prognosis are admitted, or if children are admitted after the time when they might learn best, the burdon upon professional staff and their aides is particularly heavy. Although there is a good deal to be said for separating slow moving from faster moving children, it is valuable for staff members to be able to work with both groups.

Inclusion criteria

Language unit provision will generally be for cases of developmental language disorder though some of the much smaller number of acquired cases may be taken. These do not generally include children with Landau–Kleffner syndrome who may need more medical attention than can be provided in a unit. The Landau–Kleffner syndrome is one that is acquired somewhere between the ages of 2 and 5 years. The child will have developed language but will lose it progressively, starting with verbal comprehension. The effects of this loss of comprehension on the child may be such as to suggest that he is suffering from hearing loss or behavioural disturbance but the disorder is that of auditory receptive aphasia (Robinson, 1987). Children with Landau–Kleffner syndrome are likely to have seizures and EEG examinations will show abnormal and epileptic features. The prognosis is variable. Some children recover their language function whilst others show permanent impairment with or without further seizures. The children who fail to recover language spontaneously are likely to need a protected residential environment or one which is part of a neuropaediatric unit because of the severity of the disorder and its medical implications.

ICAN guidelines have taken the step of specifying the four broad groups of language-disordered children most suited to language unit placement:

1. Children with phonological–grammatical problems. This group has been described in Chapter 5 as the phonological–syntactic group. These children are expected to constitute the majority of the language unit clientele.
2. Children who have the above problems with the accompaniment of a receptive disorder. It is suggested that only one or two children with major comprehension problems be placed in each class.
3. Children with semantic–pragmatic problems. It is suggested that only children with mild forms of this disorder be placed in units. Children with severe disorders would be better placed in a protected environment where integration with mainstream classes is not part of the programme.
4. Children with articulatory difficulties based upon impaired coordination of the fine movements required for speech.

Staffing

It is recommended that one teacher and one therapist be appointed full time to a class within a language unit. A class should consist of six to eight children. In addition there should be an assistant to the teacher or therapist and, as a resource person, an educational psychologist with special experience in developmental language disorders.

The provision of speech therapy is complicated by the fact that speech therapists have been employed by the Health Service following the recommendations of the Quirk committee in 1972. Thus they are not immediately at the disposal of the educational authorities. This dichotomy affects language-disordered children at many levels. It can result in the failure to detect subtle language disorders among the school-aged population. It can also result in the provision prescribed in a child's statement of special need failing to be carried out because the statement concerns the child's education, and speech therapy is provided from the health service budget. Among the many factors which militate against an integrated service for the language-disordered child, this administrative division is outstanding. In some districts, the goodwill and exertions of professionals keep the problems to a minimum, but no combination of goodwill and exertion is proof against sheer lack of personnel.

Statementing

Since the passing of the 1981 Education Act, each local education authority has a duty to ensure that special education provision is made for pupils who have special educational needs. This applies to children aged 2;0–

19;0 years. When a child is perceived to be in need of special provision, the local authority must arrange for a comprehensive assessment to be carried out. This assessment must be multi-disciplinary and take account of both educational and medical factors together with input from the child's parents and the psychologist. Any written advice which arises from the assessment becomes a Statement of Special Educational Need. The education authority has a legal obligation to meet this need. Where provision within the normal school is agreed to be adequate, the formal statement may be waived. This means that the child can potentially participate in the provisions of the national curriculum. Wedell (1989), writing about the application of the national curriculum to children with special needs, makes the point that in teaching pupils with a wide range of abilities, teachers need to 'match the breadth of content at any one level of the curriculum to their pupils' capacity to cope with it'. He goes on to underline the need for such children to be able to focus on the content at one level which is essential for the attainment of the next level. There is therefore a need for modification and flexibility in application. This is especially true where the learning difficulty includes language impairment.

A formal statement must be reviewed annually, whenever there is a change in circumstances or at the request of the parents. The situation has occurred many times where an assessment team has found a need for intensive speech–language therapy but the education authority is not in a position to provide it and the health authority cannot afford to do so.

Revisions to the 1981 Act have clarified the position with regard to the position of speech therapy. However, there is considerable variation in different parts of the country. The College of Speech Therapists has recently issued a position paper (1988b), which gives guidelines for speech therapists 'to ensure, as far as possible, that practices within their District allow for their full and appropriate involvement in the identification, assessment and meeting of Special Educational Needs'. It acknowledges that terminology may vary in different parts of the country but contends that general principles remain the same.

A parallel is to be found between the British statement and the US provision under Public Law 94-142: The Education for All Handicapped Children Act. This law entitled all handicapped children to have their educational needs met and not to be discriminated against by virtue of handicap. The education services to which they are legally entitled should enable them to have full equality of opportunity with their peers. Each state of the union could receive federal funds for the purpose of meeting the special needs of their handicapped children. If they failed to do so, they were liable for penalties under the law. This provision for handicapped children has now been twice revised, first to encompass preschool children and second to cover the needs of handicapped children and toddlers. The education authority or school district enters into a contract with the parents of the handicapped child to carry out an individualised education programme (IEP). This IEP is drawn up following multidisciplinary assessment if necessary, and with the full agreement of the parents. If the programme as agreed by both parties is not carried out, parents may sue the school district. If they are successful, the district must provide the services.

The IEP has thus much stronger backing than the British 'Statement' because it relates back to the Bill of Rights. It is a basic human right not to be discriminated against. Legal action is therefore the immediate recourse in the case of default. While the system has a strength that many British parents campaigning for services must envy, it does lead to an almost intolerable amount of litigation which can sour relations and slow down procedures. It can also lead to a certain amount of teaching to task since professionals having put their names to highly specified procedures do not feel free to take a more creative route, even if one presents itself. This can be a real detriment to dynamic language therapy.

Meeting the need

We must now look at how previous points about the nature of language disorders and the differentiation of clinical subtypes can be integrated into this discussion of the principles and practicalities of intervention. In all discussion of how best to help the children, we must bear in mind that their level of attainment will be determined by the extent to which they are able to use their own resources to compensate for their deficiencies. 'The extent to which a child is motivated to use whatever limited abilities he has determines his degree of success' (Wedell, 1980). We believe that if the child is developing language in an aberrant way, or if he is severely delayed, he must receive language teaching which assists this compensation and motivates him as an individual. General programmes of language development or stimulation will not be adequate or appropriate. Compensation may be assisted by building up individual language strengths, thus helping the child to find his own language-learning strategy. Alternatively it may be promoted by working away at weak features in order to strengthen them and improve the whole performance.

Teaching to strength or to weakness is a matter for individual decision. It has been our experience that when the child's overall cognitive or intellectual level is not high, teaching to weakness may prove discouraging. There is not enough language matrix to support the weak skill, and battering away at it may cause breakdown in overall function. Working through strength is a good therapeutic principle and should only be jettisoned upon very special consideration. We have little evidence to show that repeated work on, for example, auditory memory, can improve the memory. Improvement is more likely to come about through a number of compensatory strategies which arise from insight and resource.

Since we are working with developing children we must expect that the natural processes of maturation will exert their influence. The factors contributing to the language disorder will, both individually and collectively or interactively show change. It is the object of early intervention to accelerate this maturation. We may also expect to see a shift in the pattern of the disorder both as a result of therapy and because of the natural progress of the condition.

The following cases illustrate this pattern shift:

> S. was referred at 3;10 with no spoken language. Hearing was normal and comprehension as tested on the RDLS and the Peabody Picture Vocabulary Scale was on a par with chronological age. Social interaction was good and S. both responded to and initiated communication. Her speech performance was restricted to emotive jargon in which only mid-vowels and glides were noted. The only consonants were /n/, a dental /d/ and an occasional bilabial fricative. Direct stimulation produced recognisable approximations for the consonants /p/ /b/ /d/ /k/ and /g/. S. was unable to imitate a phonetic pattern and at first was also unable to imitate a vowel with intonation.
>
> During therapy, S. learned to imitate rising and falling cadences using sustained vowels. Articulatory shaping developed spontaneously during this time, but not the ability to imitate a phonetic sequence. Imitation of simple words consisting of CV combination only was achieved by 5 years. As the words were linked together by the coordinate 'and' (or a close approximation) a simple phonological system started to emerge. At 7 years, S. was enrolled in a newly opened language unit with the diagnosis of expressive aphasia, word-finding difficulty and severe articulation disorder. Her overall score on the WISC was 96, within normal range. At that time, abnormal prosody was still evident in utterances of more than three or four words. Normal prosody was demonstrated in short familiar phrases, e.g. 'I don't know'. Sequencing difficulties were still apparent during a demonstration session at 9;10 years when the unfamiliar word 'Jubilee' was rendered as 'julibill'; this was corrected only after several minutes of instruction. At that time pragmatic sophistication was apparent in the way S. handled conversation, following leads, initiating and giving new information when appropriate. Comprehension difficulties were now apparent in complex linguistic constructions, but needed to be probed for. S. was able to transfer into mainstream schooling with additional support from the speech therapist and educational

psychologist. Her reading skills were sufficiently well established to allow her to develop pleasure in reading, albeit at a somewhat unsophisticated level.

Motor sequencing skills and overall motor performance showed more evidence of abnormality during and after an adolescent growth spurt. Socially, S. tended to cling to her family and lacked assertiveness. Both social and motor skills improved considerably after a period at a residential college where she was able to receive regular physiotherapy. Residual problems centred upon spelling and pronunciation of words containing clusters of consonants. There appeared to be a link here in that spelling still lacked phonetic underpinning.

During her development and through the help received in the language unit and elsewhere, S. developed very obvious strategies to help maintain control of language. One was the recourse to scanning or abnormal prosody when essaying long utterances. By breaking up utterances into short tone units she may have been able to facilitate processing including the retrieval of phonological representations of content and function words. Striving to establish meaning was often accompanied by a regression in clarity of articulation. However, she was able to help herself by good pragmatic function. For example, after stumbling over the phrase 'physically handicapped' she said 'like in wheelchairs'. During her early years, S. presented a picture of verbal apraxia. The following characteristics were evident:

● Impaired ability to imitate at word and at sound level.
● Impaired prosody.
● Impairment of motor planning and timing.
● Impairment of monitoring.
● Impaired ability to carry out a sequence of movement, particularly at speed.

Later she showed characteristics of phonological–syntactic syndrome:

● Lack of articles, prepositions and pronouns.
● Omission of word endings.
● Faulty articulation.
● More difficulty with comprehension of language than initial performance suggested.

It is likely that the pattern shift was predominantly associated with cortical reorganisation which dictated its type, but the demands placed and the support given by her environment promoted the use of language. The combination of these attributes associated with skilled teaching encouraged mastery of language form. A crucial therapeutic procedure was the setting up of the articulatory loop. This subsystem has been shown to be involved in subvocal rehearsal and associated with memory span (Hitch and Halliday, 1983).

The second case history also shows the shift in the main features of language disorder in a young female:

> J. was born normally to a mother who had been hospitalised for 6 months during pregnancy because of hyperemesis (acute vomiting). The child had a birth weight of 6lb 2oz. Early development appeared normal. Subsequently there was mild spasticity of the right leg and delayed and unintelligible speech which was exacerbated by dysarthria. There was also sequential difficulty at word and sound level. Speech and physiotherapy were started at 3 years of age. According to outside criteria, J. was intelligible at 7;0 years, but the girl herself in a subsquent account (Byers Brown and Beveridge, 1979) suggests that her speech problems persisted until at least 8 years of age. A severe reading problem then became apparent. Unfortunately at this time, some 25 years ago, there were few facilities for helping language-disordered children and less understanding than now exists as to how to approach reading disabilities which ensued from these disorders. At 17 years of age, J. a girl of strong character and good overall intelligence had come to the following conclusion, 'I feel that as I cannot read now, I never will'. However, following full investigation and the construction of a specially designed reading programme, some gains were made. The investigation carried out by a psychologist and a speech therapist showed problems of analysis and synthesis in sound patterns, affecting both speech and spelling though the latter skill was now more conspicuously abnormal. For example 'alphabetically' became 'alphurbatilly', 'told' was 'tal', 'plod' was 'plood' and 'dyslexia', 'dislects'.
>
> The speech therapist's report also draws attention to occasional word substitutions and recall difficulties. The psychologists found clear evidence of reading/spelling disorder aggravated by years of educational difficulties. It was suggested that untimed testing be used in all examinations at the school which J. was required to take. In spite of J.'s discouragement, she was now showing a reading level which varied from 10 years to 14 years when untimed procedures were used. There were indications from this evaluation that had an earlier approach to reading been more systematically pursued, J. might have reached the stage of reading for pleasure. As it was, she passed 'O' level English in her General Certificate of Education examination and subsequently trained and

qualified as a children's nurse. However, writing of her life some 15 years later, she states, 'I don't have the inquisitive mind to pick up a piece of paper and see what is on it' and 'a book is just a load of print'. She has made the decision to avoid all reading as far as possible. 'I have the radio on all the time for news and information.' 'I try always to go to the same garage where I have memorised the instructions on how to fill up with petrol.' And as an overall policy, 'I try to put myself in situations where I know I can cope well and avoid others' but 'I know I am very dependent on other people'. The sum of characteristics of this language disorder would place it in the phonological–syntactic syndrome group. However, the spasticity and articulatory difficulties place it towards the motor end of that spectrum. J. would be one of those children with expressive difficulties allied to cerebral palsy originally described by Morley. A case study of a child with similar but more severe problems may be found in Byers Brown (1981, pp. 156–164). Initial therapy for such children tends to focus on movement control. In order to anticipate and so far as is possible prevent severe secondary disabilities, the ability to perceive and to analyse sound sequences should be promoted at the same time. Assessment of perceptuomotor skills must be carried out regularly in order to know where to place therapeutic emphasis. The shift which took place in J.'s case was from a condition of mild cerebral palsy affecting the organisation of movement to a broader condition of perceptual and linguistic deficit. The programme of intervention was not sufficiently comprehensive to prevent the severe language problem affecting a number of skills.

Interestingly although J. showed considerable resource in coping with her difficulties in the running of her life, she did not, either as a young child or subsequently, develop spontaneous strategies to assist herself in mastering sound patterns (for examples of such strategies, see Weeks 1974). Her failure to do so might at first have been due to lack of awareness of her problems and later to discouragement as to her inability to surmount them. It is possible, but by no means certain, that more helpful self-help strategies could have been stimulated by a cohesive and comprehensive intervention programme. In noting the absence of such programmes in the past, however, we must also be aware of cases where they have been instituted and have still not been able to guard against the shift in the condition or the variety of its manifestations. Reference has already been made to the brave and honest account given by Damico (1986). This case contradicts the unfortunately strong impression made by some observations, that early speech therapy may simply concentrate on polishing up the child's utterance and eliminating articulatory errors.

In the case described by Damico, there was thorough investigation of the language disorder in a child of 5;11 years. The characteristics were syntactic and semantic problems which were tackled by regular and systematic language therapy. The case was assessed and reassessed (see Chapter 6) and discharge was only carried out when gains had been shown in all the areas of deficit. Six years later, the child was referred back to the language clinician exhibiting severe behavioural and communicative disorder. Investigation showed a number of abnormal language behaviours which had been insufficiently probed earlier.

Damico gives a number of interesting reasons for the failure of initial therapy to eliminate subsequent problems. The impression produced is one of an experienced and conscientious clinician who is limited by the procedures available to him at any one time. However, we could contend that there can be no absolute safeguards against the recurrence of a language disorder since even the most inspired clinician must be limited in what he can observe and predict. We can safeguard ourselves against myopic adherence to a limited approach and alert ourselves to the limitations of the prevailing viewpoint. Teachers and therapists who have worked with language-disordered children over a long period of time tend to adopt approaches described by one of us (BBB), as 'core implicit and crisis induced' (Byers Brown, 1982). Thorough assessment and observation will show the nature of the problems and intervention procedures are then designed to help the child to compensate. As we encourage the child to grow and experiment in language, different problems or additional ones may be revealed. As we work hard with the children, we may push them to process more language elements than they can comfortably handle. There may then be regression in form or function while reorganisation takes place. The therapist or teacher will support and encourage the child and his family at times of crisis and if these periods are wisely handled further growth may result.

In developing children of otherwise good endowment, the limits of capacity and predictions of growth cannot be gauged to a nicety. Where limitations are general and profound, more protection and less pressure towards growth may be pursued. Failure to create appropriate effort in any handicapped child is likely to lead to passivity and inertia. It is possible that some of our early approaches to language intervention may have contributed to this result in the past by too little emphasis on function and interaction and too much emphasis on form. It will be interesting to see whether young language-disordered children can take on a more active, dynamic role in subsequent language teaching if they are prepared for it on the lines indicated by Aldred (1983). In this article a language group within the nursery environment is described. Emphasis throughout the activities was placed upon language in context and use. The natural social environment of the group was seen as the stimulator of language interactions with natural reinforcement being provided for successful use. The children admitted to the group received comprehensive individual assessments including analysis of a 30-minute speech sample through the LARSP and PRISM procedures (see Chapter 6). Phonology was analysed through the Grunwell model (1975) and the language functions outlined by Halliday (1975) were used as the framework for describing language use.

The children demonstrated delay in all parameters of language development. Two groups could be identified, one with predominant deficit in verbal expressive abilities and one with predominantly poor verbal receptive skills. The expressive group showed initially poor grasp of phrase structure with relatively advanced clause structure high in semantic content and relying upon information-loaded lexemes. Phonology was delayed. The receptive group showed advanced phrase structures, stereotyped clause structures and restricted semantic functions. This group showed few phonological immaturities. Children in both groups showed gains following intervention. The expressive group added to their range of linguisitic structures and the receptively impaired group improved in interpersonal communication and in the regulatory aspects of language function. All children advanced in verbal receptive skills. Aldred comments that perhaps the most important change was in their social-communication skills. The children widened the functional range of their language and actively sought to widen their own environment. This change came about through therapy which aimed to follow the child's lead and which relied upon the social interaction developed in the group to provide the primary motivator.

Parents were actively involved and became increasingly aware of the functions of language. As a natural consequence, they started to give their children increased communicative responsibility in the home. This type of management would appear to have a great deal to offer to the preschool child. It stimulates language development in a way that leaves parent and child with functional gains. It could thus provide a valuable precursor to individual therapy or to language unit placement and special teaching.

Intervention procedures in relation to specified clinical subtypes

In our discussion of intervention procedures we will follow the order indicated by our language processing model in Chapter 4.

Verbal auditory agnosia

Since this condition is characterised by inability to interpret information presented through the auditory channel, the thrust of the intervention procedure should be through the visual channel. Children who have severe auditory perceptual problems, or who show the full syndrome of verbal auditory agnosia (receptive aphasia), are candidates for special school placement. This is true for both the developmental syndrome and for the condition acquired in early childhood (Landau–Kleffner syndrome). The psychological picture is different in the acquired cases since, if children have started to make sense of the speech around them, the sudden loss of this ability will be very frightening and bewildering.

Young children may first be enrolled in individual therapy programmes while suitable educational placement is found for them. The therapist may then institute a signed system of communication which will be the basis of the child's acquisition of language structure. Several special schools in Britain have adopted the Paget–Gorman signing system and so speech therapists will use this with individual children who later may be offered places in these schools. Signing provides an interim measure to promote communication and lay down word order concept in children with less severe impairment. The Paget–Gorman signing system has been described as an important means of cueing some children in to the spoken and written word and to the conventions of word order for it is a grammatically based system. A useful paper on the need to establish criteria of measurement in signing systems is that by Faucett and Clibbons (1983). Kiernan has also written extensively on the subject of signing.

The first programme to help these children was developed by McGinnis (1963); it became established as 'the association method'. Subsequently criticised for its rigidity, it was successful in giving order and structure to communicative attempt and providing a basis for language development. The importance of a planned clear approach was effectively demonstrated and has never really been questioned since. There were several schemes which employed visual representations, e.g. Lea's Colour Pattern Scheme (Lea, 1965) to teach parts of speech and word order. Whereas the McGinnis method placed emphasis on visual representation of single sounds in order to facilitate utterance, the Lea method taught whole words. This enabled children to move on to simple written language as a means of communication while they were still unable to produce intelligible words. The question as to whether to try to generate utterance at the same time as teaching symbol representation through the visual form was in most cases influenced by the population within the various establishments. It was deemed very unlikely that some children would ever be able to produce intelligible utterances and so speech would be of no practical value to them. The present emphasis on early signing for a number of severely language-disordered children has taken the pain out of this decision. Signing is a personally expressive medium and the child may be able to combine it with speech at some later time. In some cases it is thought to facilitate spoken language. As has been stated earlier, the prognosis for these children is not good so far as creative, competent language is concerned and it is therefore doubly important to find a medium through which they can receive and express ideas.

The acquisition of signing allows aphasic adolescents to share social activities with the signing deaf, thus enlarging their circle of friends. Since they are inevitably isolated from their normal peer groups, this enlargement is important. The restrictions which the condition imposes upon their cognitive and social development means that they may remain immature and egocentric. Social contacts, shared activities with normal children and the promotion of team efforts form a very large part of the schools' activities.

The main changes in management which have come about in the 25 years since the McGinnis method was propagated are the influence of linguistic criteria upon all communication and the development of visual teaching devices through computer programs. The principle of employing visual modality methods to compensate for auditory deficits has not changed. A means must be provided that will lead to the acquisition and storage of lexical items. The conventional structure within which these items can be placed must then be taught.

Rapin and Allen point out that the population of children with verbal auditory agnosia will include children who have autistic features and are profoundly retarded intellectually. Such children are unable to acquire language through a grammatically based signing system, though they may fare better with an iconic method like MAKATON. In the present state of our knowledge, however, to be realistic, we do not have much to offer them beyond general care. In their discussion of auditory agnosia, Rapin and Allen subscribe to the view that this receptive syndrome (without autism) is a 'pure' syndrome with severe consequences for language processing including production. We would agree with this view since these children suffer by order of magnitude when compared with those who have comprehension difficulties when faced with continuous language. The children with verbal auditory agnosia do not understand some auditory sequences and misunderstand others. The auditory channel is not useful to them as a means of learning. Fortunately, the condition is rare. However, our discussion of language processing models draws attention to the possible subcategories of comprehension impairment that can be found at an early age. If some very young children do show comprehension deficits without the full syndrome of verbal auditory agnosia, it is essential that their auditory decoding abilities be developed. Carefully graded auditory and verbal stimulation is the route indicated.

Semantic–pragmatic disorder

We agree with the position taken by Bishop and Rosenbloom (1987) that we have here a range of conditions rather than one syndrome. This may be briefly exemplified by contrasting the following case with that of the child F. given in Chapter 5.

> A. was first seen at the age of 4;0 years. He had shown normal developmental milestones following an induced birth at 31 weeks due to maternal hypertension. Forceps were employed and there was a delay in onset of respiration.
>
> At the time of his referral, his expressive language was fluent but with some syntactic errors. Some echoic speech was evident. Responses to comprehension items on the RDLS were inconsistent. An overall score of 2;3 years was obtained. He indulged in a considerable amount of monologue during play.
>
> Fine motor control was poor.
>
> During assessment he showed distractability and other attentional difficulties.
>
> A. showed 'unusual and phenomenal skill at reading'. He could read complex instructions at sight (e.g. the psychologist's test sheet) but without understanding. At one point, he scored 170 on the Schonell graded reading test. These attributes place him in the category of 'hyperlexic children'. He was subsequently diagnosed as autistic. However, after 2 years in a special nursery group he was transferred to a mainstream primary class. He continued to show conceptual–semantic problems. Although he had some difficulty in forming relationships with other people he could no longer be considered autistic.

Both A. and F. showed well developed syntactic and phonological skills but their expressive language was inappropriate to the situations they were in or to the people they were with. However A. had the special feature of his reading skill and showed sufficient signs of autistic behaviour to be so classified for a period of his development. The diagnosis of autism was never considered in F.'s case.

In discussing semantic–pragmatic disorders, we do not wish to become too involved in the present controversy as to whether or not such behaviour is always associated with autism. We expect to see less extreme views being propagated as more information becomes available. Many speech therapists' opposition to the possibility that some of their language-disordered children are autistic is based on faulty understanding of the changing nature of autism. It is not always appreciated that autistic children improve and develop over time. As they do so, different manifestations of their autism become more or less dominant. Autism, like language disorder, is not an absolute state within which no change is to be expected. Children with semantic–pragmatic disorders of language may show autistic features and children who are autistic will have difficulty with semantic–pragmatic aspects of language. We suggest that the decision as to who should work with them be based upon which professional has most to offer the child at any particular period of his development and there is also ample opportunity for joint work between teachers, psychologists and speech therapists. Since we are now in a position to define and assess the language disorders which children with autistic features may show, it is logical and humane to develop programmes of language therapy for them.

We would therefore like to make a number of points in relation to intervention for children with semantic–pragmatic disorders. These children typically show a lack of interest in interacting with other people. Some of them are very unresponsive during early childhood and give the impression of general cognitive delay. 'He was difficult to stimulate and difficult to communicate with. He would sit in his pushchair like a little doll paying little attention to activities around him.' Present thinking will therefore encourage the development of interaction between the child and others. While this is extremely important, we believe it should be handled with care. During their early development, the children may need some protection from the battering of an environment, much of which they cannot understand. Continual pressure towards interaction will be fatiguing and could be harmful.

Throughout therapy and education, emphasis should be on the semantic aspect of the condition. These children are unable to appreciate the contextual significance of words. Thus they have comprehension deficits which are testable and functional problems that are continually revealed.

> 'When he was six he started in infant school. The headmistress did not understand his problem. She told him once to pick up litter. He did so but did not put it in the bin. He found it hard to follow even simple instructions and could not follow them through to their logical conclusion. Each day, on the way to school we practised saying "Please tell me again slowly". He still makes the same request at sixteen.'

One other brief illustration reminds us of the impossibility of teaching every language nuance. Mother: 'Oh, the alarm's gone off.' Child: 'No, It's gone on'.

Intervention must first attempt to develop simple comprehension through the use of speech in function. Requests for actions rather than for speech should be made. Activities should next be introduced in which the child can use simple speech to direct the adult. Some suggestions may be found in Warner, Byers Brown and McCartney (1984). Throughout the early stages of intervention an attempt to avoid giving ammunition for further semantic–pragmatic manifestations should be made. Thus talking too much and at a level above the child's understanding should be avoided. This will only encourage inattention. Modelling should only be used when the utterance is clearly related to an activity that the child can understand. Otherwise only further stereotyped utterance is being encouraged. Simple labelling should be discouraged. F. when shown a picture of a house immediately launched into a catalogue of 'That's a window, that's a door, that's a chimney' etc. without being able to say anything about their function. Word meanings should not be assumed to have been absorbed after one demonstration. They must be continually used and demonstrated in a functional manner employing different situations, rather in the manner described for criterion-referenced assessments in Chapter 6. If the child is able to tolerate, then enjoy interactions, he may be introduced into a small group programme such as they described by Aldred (1983). The functional communicative aspect of language can be reinforced, leaving the therapist or teacher individual time to work on word meanings.

The child must still be encouraged to take an active part and here a metalinguistic approach may be very helpful in reinforcing semantic aspects. For example, he may draw a 'big' man, sitting in the 'big' chair or give Mummy a 'big' kiss. This working and reworking of words in context is one of the most important features of intervention and is one which will continue throughout education, making use of reading and writing as well as speech. It involves teaching the child to 'know' about language. These children have strengths in motor planning and execution and also in some aspects of auditory processing since their speech is clear and intelligible. In order to convert these strengths into assets they need systematic teaching to support their weaknesses at the following levels:

● Conceptual level: intention to speak, appreciation of turn taking, symbol acquisition.
● Abstract level: semantic appreciation, recognition and memory, creation of functional language structures.
● Auditory/receptive level: ability to relate incoming information to meaningful concepts.
● Linguistic level: application of linguistic rules deduced through generalisation.
● Feedback circuits: regulation of behaviour, self-monitoring.

A central constituent of intervention lies, therefore, in the cognitive domain. The semantically and pragmatically impaired child presents a complex picture of cognitive deficit. Stimulation of thought processes must proceed concurrently with the teaching of language form and function. Assistance in constructing teaching procedures may therefore be gleaned from texts about children's thought as well as from classic language pathology texts (Wiig and Semel, 1980; Wiig, 1987).

Although it is important not to capitalise and overpromote phenomena such as reading without understanding (barking at print), it is very important to cultivate genuine talents.

'At the age of eight he began recorder lessons. He could not read music but enjoyed making a noise and "played" in assembly with the group. I taught him to mime. He just had to watch the other children and follow their lead.'

Then 'At nine years he began flute lessons with an old student friend who knew about his problems. As there were only two flautists in the junior school he became a "star", in his own eyes anyway. Self esteem causes a person to grow and his natural talent began to show. His flute became his means of communicating his feelings and he plays with great sensitivity.'

Today this boy (aged 16) is a member of his local youth orchestra and choir. He plays the piano and the piccolo in addition to the flute. He has passed seven subjects in his General Certificate of Education examination and is to take music and another subject at 'A' level. His written language is still 'chatty' and unstructured, but he is very strongly motivated to improve. He had a very severe semantic–pragmatic problem in childhood and his improvement is due to a combination of inspired and loving home support and strong self-motivation. His parents were told when he was 2 years of age that he was severely subnormal 'with no meaningful future'.

Verbal dyspraxia

Although the most salient presenting feature in verbal dyspraxia may be the articulatory/phonological deficit, we have found from clinical experience that this is not a fruitful level at which to begin a programme of intervention. Perhaps reasons for this will become clear when the features which characterise developmental dyspraxic disorders are considered. The description given in Chapter 5 included two major points, the first being that this is not a unitary disorder but that rather in the same way that the semantic–pragmatic disorder occurs on a continuum of severity so is it the case with developmental verbal dyspraxia (DVD) (Crary, 1984). Some types of the disorder appear to derive from higher order linguistic processing (i.e. they are more 'aphasic' in nature) and others resemble errors in motor processing (i.e. they are more 'dysarthric'). The second point made in the description was that because of incomplete language development in children the disorder is more likely to manifest itself as being predominantly linguistically determined.

There are two broadly connected areas on which intervention must be focused. These are:

1. Non-segmental aspects.
2. Segmental aspects.

We consider it essential to begin with the first. Developmentally this seems to make sense, for non-segmental aspects of language are both understood and produced before segmental forms. Furthermore, as was described in Chapter 4, linguistic processing of prosodic features probably takes place well upstream in the production chain. Prosodic disorders are therefore seen as an intrinsic part of DVD and not as overlaid features resulting from a primary motor deficit. Byers Brown and Lewis (1984) and Byers Brown (1988) (and also in this text, p. 77) have drawn attention to a group of children who showed a preference for vowel sequences /uh uh uh/ which they used referentially and with variation in volume. It was suggested that this was a communicative strategy adopted by the children who had not yet developed adequate motor schemata.

In planning remediation one needs to consider the components of prosody, the tone-group, tone and tonicity. Additionally stress, rhythm and pause are important. Twelve out of the 13 children in the Edwards' pilot study (1982) showed difficulties in signalling change in stress, rhythm and intonation. Their response in assessment tasks where a change of stress indicated a change of meaning tended towards syllabic type speech with equal and even stress.

It is probably best to begin with a general rhythmic programme by making the child aware of the properties of prosody. This can be undertaken by the use of rhymes and jingles. Not only is it necessary to aim for rhythmic production, but the appreciation of changes in pitch direction and in stress patterns is also very important. The child needs to listen to demonstrations of change and to be able to identify their nature. Since many of these children have an *associated* motor problem (clumsiness) it may be fruitful to gradually introduce a rhythmic motor activity concomitantly with the language work. Tapping movements which accompany speech are sometimes useful, but this should be self-generated and not imposed by an outside source like a metronome. It is stressed that there is not a cause–effect relationship between movement difficulties and DVD. Motor programmes for each are separately determined.

Visual cues may be very helpful. For older children, writing out phrases with indication of stress and pitch change is one way of doing this. For younger children, Kellett has developed a colour scheme using blocks; for example the change in pitch direction is demonstrated by placing the 'nuclear stress' block at a higher level in a row representing the utterance. Visispeech also offers both a model and feedback. Mirror work is sometimes suggested, but our own experience of this has been very unsatisfactory. In one case it produced such frustration in a child that he broke down completely and spat at his own image.

Segmental speech problems require an approach different from that which might be adopted for an articulatory disorder. The overall emphasis is on sequence rather than on individual sounds. DVD is characterised by sequential errors which may be anticipatory, perseverative or metathetic. There is therefore little point in concentrating on sound production for it is not a case of inability to produce, but rather one where the ordering of sounds constitutes the main problem. If there is a good foundation of work on establishing normal prosodic patterns, there will already be a framework into which sequences can be slotted. Rosenbek (1974) advocates reduplicating syllable sequences using CV combinations which the child already finds relatively easy to produce. The emphasis is on slowness, and on self-monitoring. He suggests a mix of nonsense sounds and real words, the former being favoured at first since they obviate the recurrence of previous learning errors. Babbling exercises as such are not thought to be useful, for in fact they only succeed in taking the child back to a much earlier stage of development and the relationship of babbling to subsequent language is in any case not a straightforward one.

Also we do not see much value in exercises of articulatory organs. In the first place they serve no functional neurophysiological purpose in relation to speech and, secondly, it is generally agreed that the best way to improve speech is by speaking.

Reference has already been made to concomitant syntactic disorders. The work of Panagos, Quine and Klich (1979) has shown the close interrelationship which exists on a two-way basis between phonological and syntactic complexity. The explanation of reduced syntax through an economy of effort strategy really is untenable. It should therefore be borne in mind that there is a need to balance the two aspects, i.e. when working at phonological level to resort to uncomplicated syntactic forms and vice versa.

Auditory discrimination work *per se* has yielded disappointing results (Yoss and Darley, 1974b).

Associated problems

Reading and writing problems of a nature somewhat similar to those of speech frequently occur. This is hardly surprising for, covertly, spoken and written language may share a common processing system. Stackhouse (1982, 1985) has carried out a series of studies examining the nature of reading and spelling deficits in dyspraxic children. She found the errors to be qualitatively different from those attributable to a disorder which was predominantly phonetic in nature. Commenting on the diversity and idiosyncracy of the errors she considers that this may be an indication of different subgroups of the disorder.

The close link between the disorder of spoken and written language obviously calls for very close cooperative work between teachers and therapists so that a common strategy may be determined. Failure to do this could result in even greater confusion for a child who may already be very frustrated.

Where the disorder is very severe, placement in a language unit is highly desirable. In this way joint work can be carried out more satisfactorily.

There is also a better opportunity to pace the amount of work. Over-intensity of input can be deleterious in that it may exacerbate perseverative tendencies.

Phonological–syntactic syndrome

It has been pointed out several times that this is the largest of the clinical subgroups of language disorder. It is the one which is most likely to constitute the bulk of the language unit population. However, we must be aware of circular arguments. Although it qualifies for that position by numerical representation, it also qualifies by reason of suitability. The consensus of opinion seems to be that these children may safely be admitted to units or looked after in the mainstream school because their comprehension is sufficiently developed to allow them to understand what is going on. They do not need the protection of a special school unless their difficulties are extremely severe and/or compounded by other factors.

Children with phonological–syntactic problems may first present with delayed speech. If they are still very young, prophylactic measures may be instituted (see Chapter 3). It is desirable that the therapist study the child and monitor his progress over a period of time in order to obtain some idea of his rate of growth. Certain principles of phonology, syntax and semantics may be absorbed and acted upon during these early years. Attention may be controlled and fostered on the lines described by Cooper, Moodley and Reynell (1978). It was suggested (Byers Brown, 1971) that during this period it might be possible to observe whether the child was developing a linguistic system in a fragmented manner, or whether it was cohesive but constrained. Intervention will therefore be carried out to help the child either to organise his system or to expand it.

During the preschool years changes may occur in either direction. For example, attention may improve or attentional difficulties may remain and show increased relationship to general cognitive impairment. Motor skills may improve or there may be a gradual revelation of subtle coordination difficulties. There may be improvement in ability to generate words in order, but continued difficulty in phonological planning leading to unintelligibility. We have already drawn attention to the finding by Bishop and Edmundson (1987) that the more areas involved the poorer the prognosis. Any or all of the following areas of deficit may be found. At linguistic level: phonological representation, storage and retrieval; creation of planning frame; insertion of phonological forms into planning frame; generation and retrieval of specific linguistic forms; application of phonetic rules. At motor level: retrieval of appropriate motor schemata; generation of neuromuscular programme; articulatory presentation. Feedback circuits; feedforward of auditory and motor information to allow planning; feedback via proprioception.

The following case history indicates how some of the impairments at different levels become apparent during development.

I. was referred at 2;0 years because of the absence of words. Auditory acuity and middle ear function were normal and there was no delay in any other parameters of development. Speech–sound behaviour consisted of jargon, vowels with intonation and vocables. This would be considered normal for a child of around 12 months. A programme of language stimulation and parent guidance (in which both parents took part) was instituted. During the next 18 months I. suffered several episodes of otitis media raising the question as to whether or not this could have been a factor contributing to his speech delay. Although his hearing was normal when tested there is no guarantee that this was always the case. However, as his parents were alert to the possibility of fluctuating hearing loss and brought him regularly for assessment, it was considered an unlikely contributor to language delay.

At 3;8 I. showed a language comprehension age of 3;5 and an expressive age of 2;4 years. The overall pattern was one of slow growth. However, he had made expressive gains of about 16 months in a 20-month period. In order to determine whether this was a resolving delay or a disorder the pattern of language development must be looked at. The following characteristics were noted: high proportion of nouns in relation to other words, telegraphic utterances, failure to observe word boundaries, late emergence of phonological system, continuing use of gesture. Intervention accordingly shifted to a solid programme of language building, learning new words, memorising rhymes and word games, the child giving word directives and listening to stories read by the mother or therapist in order to retell them. I. was able to manage in normal primary school with therapy support and appeared to be functioning normally when he entered junior school. No educational difficulties were reported. It seems likely that I.'s difficulties were at the linguistic level, particularly affecting planning. This appeared to be strengthened by the measures taken. I. never showed pragmatic difficulties. His good cognitive ability was demonstrated in his progress and was always apparent to his parents. (Father's comment: 'He could buy and sell his elder brother!'.)

Early therapy should provide the young language-delayed child with more information or help him to organise the information he possesses. It attempts to guide him through the stages of progressive differentiation and make the right choices at the right time. The therapist must therefore be aware of the features which she is attempting to control or modify. What are the language units which the child is producing and which he appears able to handle? What units does he need to round out his system? Will he be able to deduce rules for himself if stimulated by simple speech which is interesting to him and which contains considerable repetition and redundancy? Or, does he need to be taught a few discriminations in a direct manner? Such information can well be learned through interacting with the child in a simple natural manner that will allow him to converse. This will show how much he is able to follow the lead of an adult speaker, to pattern his speech upon that of the therapist and to experiment with speech and language forms.

Recent research (Bishop, 1983, 1987b; Duxbury, 1986; Van der Lely and Dewart, 1986) has now revealed that children with such disorders may be suffering from subtle deficits of comprehension which only become apparent as the language to which they are exposed becomes more complex (see also the discussion of R. as cited in Chapter 5). This may be checked by steady reappraisal and reassessment of the child's functional levels. However, although these children may have passed earlier assessment tests at appropriate levels, functional comprehension difficulty is observed frequently by the therapist. As one becomes familiar with the child's personality and overall behaviour, one develops greater sensitivity to even slight changes. A delay in response or momentary confusion will signal lack of comprehension and this may be tackled immediately. If the mother is present (and in the case of individual therapy this is extremely likely), advice may be given as to how to deal with such signs when they are observed at home.

Gibson and Ingram (1983), in a diary account of the development of comprehension and production in a language-delayed child over a period of 17 months, provide valuable information about changes which took place. Progress was characterised by a series of spurts which coincided with changes in developmental milestones. The authors suggest that this might be one way in which clinicians can capitalise on normal growth to stimulate progress in language.

Within the considerable span of this clinical subtype there can be a wide range of symptoms and signs and, of course, severity. Children who are identified at the stage of language delay may be well documented by the time they reach 5;0 years of age. The rate of their progress, its even or uneven nature and the factors which appear to influence it may be helpfully described. It should be becoming apparent whether the child is going to manage within the normal school or whether he will need provision in a unit or in a special school. Concurrent with this will be the decision to embark on a teaching programme based upon the child's individual language profile. Such a profile may be derived from the measures described by Aldred or may emerge through the procedures associated with recognised language schemes. The popularity of the

Derbyshire Language Scheme (Masidlover and Knowles, 1982) testifies to the need that units have to make use of some developed scheme. Other children may be considered suitable candidates for the highly structured methods advised by Hutt (1986) and propagated through ICAN. Such decisions are made in accordance with the avowed policy of unit or school as well as in the interests of individual children.

The present weight of evidence seems to show that it is unwise to embark on a structured scheme before the child has been observed and worked with over a period of time and during the early developmental period. If he is a late referral or a very severe case, he may merit special consideration. Harris's (1984) valuable discussion is likely to remain particularly pertinent to all questions of this kind.

Lexical–syntactic deficit

German (1985, 1987) has studied this deficit extensively as also have Wiig and Semel (1984) and Wiig and Becker-Caplan (1984). It is a disorder which may not be readily apparent. The child may be thought of as being quiet and non-communicative because of the sparseness of spoken language. In contrast to the quiet children there are those who appear to be almost garrulous with a near incessant flow of talk. Both types require careful investigation so that appropriate remediation can be undertaken. In the first instance a combination of formal testing (e.g. German, 1986) and analysis of a spontaneous sample of speech may help to identify certain classes of words which present difficulties of retrieval for the child. In the second case, it is likely that closer investigation of spontaneous speech will reveal a fair amount of emptiness. This needs to be viewed very carefully for we are all prone to use filler pauses and it was pointed out in Chapter 4 that these 'non-fluencies' probably signify stretches of active planning of speech. But abnormality is indicated by the amount of meaningless insertions which usually precede content words. (Crystal (1981) incidentally calls into question definitions of and distinctions between content and function words.) Typical of this emptiness is 'Well...Well we went to this kind of er place and then we we put on these things and we sort of we played this game.' (This represents an account of going to another school to play football.)

Speech is characterised by revision, by repair and by obvious searches for the word. Interestingly the same phenomenon is apparent in the speech of many normal elderly people, although here it is concentrated more specifically on names. We have made reference to syntagmatic and paradigmatic associations which occur in a developmental sequence. This factor needs to be borne in mind in planning remedial work as do other categorisations.

The aims of remedial work are to enlarge the child's 'internal dictionary' and to build up associative networks which facilitate access to vocabulary.

Crystal (1981, p. 147) outlines a classification of paradigmatic relations based on Lyons' (1977) work. He emphasises the need to consider context in relation to classification. The classes he lists are as follows.

Synonomy

He points out that it may not be helpful to ask the child to find a word 'the same as....' unless a context is provided. For example, a synonym of the word 'wicked' might be 'bad' but there are instances where the two are not interchangeable, viz. weather, rotteness, health. To avoid this the word retrieval task should always be framed in a sentence. 'King John was a bad king. Tell me another word for *bad.*'

Opposition

This includes antonymy where there is a binary contrast: long/short; in/out. Crystal describes further subcategories of oppositeness which merit study, but in the present outline of intervention procedures these are inappropriate.

Hyponomy

This is where one encounters superordinate and subordinate relations. For example, 'vegetable' is a superordinate category. Subordinates are 'potato, carrot, peas, leeks' etc.

Israel (1984) provides some very useful procedures to facilitate word retrieval. These include superordinate, subordinate associations as above:

> A pigeon is a — , Blackbirds, robins swans are all — , An apple is a fruit.
> Which of the following are fruits? Grape, orange, cake....
> Parts of the body naming.
> Similarities.
> Syntagmatic associations.
> Tell me all the words you can think of when I say — Teddy.

Both cueing techniques, i.e. providing associated clues, and recall as in games like Kim's game are valuable in facilitating retrieval.

Wiig and Semel (1980) have described detailed procedures for treating lexical–syntactic deficits.

While syntax obviously features in this deficit, it does also seem to encompass a sizeable semantic component. It is possible that restricted syntax is an outcome of the word-finding difficulty.

Unless the condition is very severe or is associated with other deficits as was the case with the child R. whose primary problem was a phonological–syntactic deficit (Chapter 5), children who have this disorder will be treated routinely within health service settings. Close cooperation with teaching staff for purposes of guidance and reinforcement is essential.

Phonological deficits

It is not proposed to describe intervention here, for the emphasis throughout the description of language disorders has focused on syndromes. Moreover, it has been shown that in the majority of cases, phonological disorders occur in conjunction with deficits at other levels. That is not to say that they do not merit specialised intervention; on the contrary the amount of detail required in analysis and planning of treatment precludes a description in this text.

We can do no better than to advise the reader to refer to the following texts: Grunwell (1981, 1982a), Dean and Howell (1986), Howell and Dean (1987), Hill, Howell and Walters (1988), Howell and McCartney (1989). The last four groups of authors advocate a metalinguistic approach to therapy. Reference to metalinguistics has been made throughout this text either explicitly or implicitly when we have sought to emphasise the child's role in the remediation of his language. Van Kleek (1981) considers that the functions of metalinguistic skills have considerable value in clinical application. They offer a framework in which to differentiate between deficits that may be either linguistic or metalinguistic in origin. Therapy tasks sometimes require a child to reflect on a language he does not yet know. Such a situation may occur in very rigidly designed language programmes. Van Kleek parallels the development of metalinguistic awareness with a Piagetian model. In the case of young children (up to age 6 or 7 years) this is the preoperational phase. At this stage children are able to focus on only one aspect of the linguistic code at a time. Semantic awareness precedes that of syntax. Stackhouse (1975) in a discussion of differences between phonological and phonetic disorders draws attention to the value of the child being taught to recognise the properties of the language which he finds difficult to reproduce.

Throughout this chapter, we have considered types of intervention which the speech therapist may utilise; in other words, we have focused on methodological aspects, the speech therapy process. An equally important feature which has a significant contribution to make to the success of the therapeutic endeavour is the dyadic relationship between child and therapist. More recently there has been a focus on this sociolinguistic aspect (e.g. Letts, 1985). Ripich and Panagos (1985), Panagos, Bobkoff and Scott (1986), Panagos et al. (1988) have employed discourse theory to analyse clinical procedures. This they have applied to both verbal and non-verbal interaction. The clinical session is divided into lesson, task and remedial sequence. Under the first heading is included the opening phase when greetings are exchanged, questions are asked about progress etc. The work phase concentrates on the task in hand for the current session and the closing phase includes reminders, future plans and farewell greetings. The task phase begins with instructions and illustrations, then moves on to the actual procedures and is finalised by discussion of the next steps to be taken in the process of therapy. The remedial sequence relates to actual therapeutic techniques, the request for a particular response and the evaluation of that response. For many clinicians, this is a familiar routine which is adopted subconsciously. Nevertheless an analysis of interactive elements may be helpful in revealing reasons for specific failures and successes in therapy.

Chapter 8
Reflection and Future Developments

Summary

This chapter considers the feasibility of devising a classification of language disorders. Problems and confusions of terminology are discussed. Different types of taxonomies are described, in the context of a general review of the aims and content of the text. As well as a retrospective view, current and future trends in speech therapy are suggested.

In the management of language disordes there is a logical progression which has to be followed. Assessment will lead to diagnosis and this in turn should enable the particular type of disability to be assigned to a category within a classificatory scheme. As well as the progressive element, there is also an interactionary aspect, for the classification must have originally derived from the results of assessment procedures. Closely linked to classification of terminology, Chapter 1 has at the outset stated some of the problems surrounding this issue, in the review of the plethora of labels which have come to represent somewhat similar types of disorder. The title of this text, in fact, serves to illustrate the dilemma of 'How shall a thing be called?'. The problem has its origin partly in history for much of the early work undertaken by speech therapists was firmly rooted in a medical model and particularly in that of those traditionally arch taxonomists, the neurologists. Terminology therefore followed very much the pattern of Graeco-Latin derivation. Edwards (1985) referring to various attempts made by the College of Speech Therapists to revise and update the terminology remarked that the task had 'become so Sisyphean that it now seems unlikely that anything resembling an extended version of the original will ever be printed'. The futility of this undertaking parallels well with poor Sisyphus's frustrations.

Types of classification

The three types of classification most commonly encountered are (Nation and Aram, 1977):

1. Aetiological.
2. Behavioural.
3. Process based.

Aetiological

This is based on a traditional medical model in which the disorder is defined by its cause. A very obvious one would be *developmental dysphasia* which has an immediate neurological connotation. But the value of such a classification is limited for it tells the investigator little about the language of the child. In fact this particular term can only really be defined by what it is not: not deaf, not mentally handicapped, not behaviourally disturbed etc. It is therefore a perilous undertaking to place reliance on this as the only form of taxonomy, for it alone will not give any very clear indication of the nature of the language disorder. The imprecision of this type of classification has led to the considerable difficulties associated with epidemiological surveys as has been discussed (Chapter 1).

Another limitation of a purely aetiologically based taxonomy is that developmental language disorders are not unitary. We have described the term as encompassing a whole range of loosely connected conditions any of which may arise from a different aetiology. Genetic, chromosomal, atypical lateralisation and focal factors have all been cited and in each case these putative causes have been supported by evidence from published studies. Used in conjunction with other classification systems, this model can be of value and as long as speech therapy continues to have affiliation to medicine, at least within the National Health Service, then a working knowledge of this taxonomy is useful in communication with medical colleagues.

Behavioural

From this concentration on aetiology, there was a shift in the 1960s towards a concern with describing language behaviour. This was the direct result of the influence of linguistics for it was during this period that there was a marked incursion of linguists into the domain of language pathology with most fruitful results. Their work led to a preoccupation with descriptive data, and published studies during this decade are characteristically full of immensely detailed breakdowns of language behaviour. However, it gradually became apparent that description of itself provided an insubstantial basis from which a full understanding of the nature of language disorders might be found. Marshall (1983) writes': 'If we could link (normative) functional representations with their anatomico-physiological realization in a *principled* [author's italics] fashion, we would be able to understand the effect of differentially placed lesions in an *explanatory* [our italics] rather than merely *descriptive* [our italics] mode.' This quotation refers to acquired disorders; how much greater therefore is the problem of finding explanations for developmental conditions.

In the last 10 years or so, behavioural models of classification have extended their fields of interest to include interactive aspects of language. The growth of pragmatics as we have seen has undoubtedly been responsible for this and stemming from the early work of Halliday and of others, particularly Bates, systems of assessment and classification have evolved. Linguists have also moved away from a concern with discrete levels of language and have been quick to recognise the relationship between these. This is apparent in the terminology we have used throughout the book for clinicians have long been aware of the interstratified nature of these levels.

Process-based model

The third type of classification, the *process-based* model, attempts both description and explanation. It includes cognitive and linguistic factors as well as a consideration of possible neurological correlates of language pathology. Chapter 4 in reviewing language processing has endeavoured to address this tripartite involvement and the ensuing description of subtypes of language disorder has illustrated the application of these models. It is possibly this third model of classification which best fits with current assessment procedures described in Chapter 6. For example, a careful analysis of language production may be able to reveal the level of processing at which breakdown or failure occurs. Is the deficit of a higher

Table 8.1 Three classifications of language disorder

Aetiological	*Behavioural*	*Process-based*
Receptive aphasia Central auditory dysfunction	Limited expressive language Semantic disability	Auditory imperception Failure to access semantic memory Limited production
Expressive aphasia (Broca type)	Word-finding difficulty Syntactic limitation Phonological–prosodic disability	Phonological–syntactic disorder Some comprehension problems Impaired connection between higher order schemata of linguistic units and peripheral motor planning

order nature in terms of retrieval and/or selection of phonological elements, or does it relate to more peripheral aspects with aberrant phonetic features, or does it manifest signs of both? These are the sort of questions that clinicians need to ask, for the result of such analysis is crucial in the planning of effective remediation.

Table 8.1 provides an illustration of the way in which each of the three taxonomies might include two specific types of language disorder.

Delayed and disordered language

A differentiation between these terms has proved to be the focus for a considerable amount of work and this has been fully discussed in earlier chapters. To date there does not appear to be any consensus as to clear definitions which might distinguish them, but this is not an indication of failure. Rather it serves to emphasise the continuum nature of language which has been a recurring theme throughout the text. Extremes are relatively easy to identify and Crystal in 1980 provides examples at different linguistic levels. But he then goes on to point out that in many cases there is no clear-cut evidence; language delay is on a gradient which moves towards disorder. Obviously, it is essential that the child's language should be seen in the context of other development and much of the current thinking which has been cited here places great emphasis on discrepancies between overall level of language development and overall level of cognitive development. Another important aspect is that of age. We know that stages of language acquisition are not immutable; we also observe that children employ differing strategies to reach them. However, there does seem to be some agreement that the third year is the time when systematic investigation may differentiate between delay and disorder. Before that, decisions are likely to be more tentative in the light of present knowledge.

One intention of this final chapter was to consider whether a firm taxonomy of developmental language disorder is a realistic possibility. The progression of our ideas with the growth of the writing leads us to think that this is not the most fruitful way at the present time towards furthering knowledge. Descriptions of early language development, prophylactic measures, the gradual shading of immature language into full blown disorder all serve to confirm the notion of language and language disorder being on a continuum ranging from normality through to deviance. Within the categories of deviance too we have not found it helpful to regard them as discrete entities for they share commonalities. Language as one of the most complex aspects of human behaviour does not readily lend itself to strict taxonomy. It seems therefore that labels will always have to be accompanied by description and by explanation if remediation is to meet with success. One of the chief values of a classification system is that, having identified a particular type of disorder, we should then be in a strong position to recommend the most suitable type of intervention. We have considered this in the light of available resources at the present time.

As our ability to identify particular types of language disorder grows, we may hope to seek out the specific components of these disorders within other populations of handicapped children. In this text, the emphasis has been on these children for whom language disorder is the essential handicap. We know that it may also occur in children who are intellectually impaired, hearing impaired or who have cerebral palsies. Such children will need a combination of intervention approaches to assist them to cope with their combined handicaps. As we gain more assurance in the area of intervention for language disorder, we must ensure that the needs of multiply handicapped children are met.

The views we have expressed regarding the nature of language disorders coupled with the likelihood that resources will show little appreciable growth in the immediate future give cause for a consideration, albeit speculative, about the direction speech therapy may follow within the next decade. We are aware that change is taking place, though there are still signs of adherence to the well worn pattern of once-weekly, one-to-one sessions as a matter of expediency rather than because the needs of a particular child favour that type of intervention.

At the heart of such change we see a need for radical reappraisal of selection criteria. Allied to this is the need for speech therapists to identify the nature of their specific knowledge and skills, i.e. those which are unique to them and not shared with parallel professional workers.

There are undoubtedly many language-disordered children who will derive the greatest benefit from cooperative work with teachers and to this end the indications of development of shared knowledge which have been described here are most welcome.

Likewise the active involvement of parents in remedial work is also likely to be fruitful, particularly so with children who have moderately severe language disorders.

There still, however, remains a core of children with intractable impairment who require concentrated specialised help which will involve the therapist in detailed planning and which will call upon a unique combination of knowledge derived from developmental psychology, neurobiological development and from applied linguistic science. For such children, rigid adherence to a pre-packaged language programme is unlikely to be helpful, for the intervention must be individually planned. The main advantage of such programmes is that, provided they are not over-prescriptive, they offer a common meeting ground and a guideline for cooperative effort between therapists and others. Over the last decade or so there has been a shift of focus on to those aspects of language which are more particularly concerned with communication and this is welcome. But our enthusiasm for pragmatic proficiency should not make us overlook the fact that those children with severe language disorder have no tools with which to demonstrate their ability to use language. For these, work must begin at the 'coal face' of structure and meaning. It is in this sphere that we consider speech therapists to possess special expertise.

A redistribution of work therefore seems to be a possibility in the future and indeed there are already signs that this is taking place. In relation to developmental language disorders there seem to be three main areas in which speech therapists' work will develop to a much greater extent.

In the first instance there needs to be a concentration and application of therapeutic skills for the benefit of severely language-disordered children.

Cooperative work with parents both in devising and monitoring their work must be encouraged to a much greater extent.

Thirdly, we need to be aware of the special contribution which teachers are able to make especially in those cases where learning difficulties and language problems coexist. To this end teachers must have the opportunity to learn about the nature of disordered language while therapists in turn also need to become more familiar with the ways in which teachers seek to help those with learning difficulties. But precisely because there is much current uncertainty and ever greater discovery still to be made in the future about the nature of language disorders, we strongly advocate a flexible approach. Knowledge accrues as more research is carried out; a book on this subject written 10 years ago would have differed substantially from the present text, just as one which may be written 10 years hence will reflect new thoughts and views. That is no bad thing for how else could progress come about.

References

AFASIC (1988). *Language Unit Guidelines* 347. Central Markets, London EC1 9NH

ALDRED, C. (1983). Language in use. *Bulletin of College of Speech Therapists,* October

ALLEN, G.D. and HAWKINS, S. (1978). The development of phonological rhythm. In: *Syllables and Segments,* A. Bell and J.D. Hooper (Eds), Amsterdam: North Holland.

ARAM, D. and NATION, J. (1975). Patterns of language behavior in children with developmental language disorders. *J. Speech Hear. Res.* **18**, 229–241.

ARAM, D. and NATION, J. (1980). Preschool language disorders and subsequent language and academic difficulties. *J. Commun. Dis.* **13**, 159–170.

ARAM D. and NATION, J. (1982). *Child Language Disorders,* St Louis: C.V. Mosby.

ARAM, D., EKELMAN, B. and NATION, J. (1984). Preschoolers with language disorders. Ten years later. *J. Speech Hear. Res.* **27**, 244–282.

ARBIB, M.A. (1972). *The Metaphorical Brain.* New York: Wiley.

BAKER, LEA (1988). The use of language sample analysis. *Bulletin of College of Speech Therapists,* London, May

BARTAK, L. RUTTER, M. and COX, A. (1975). A comparative study of infantile autism and specific developmental language disorders *Br. J. Psychiat.* **126**, 127–145.

BATH, D. (1981). Developing the speech therapy service in day nurseries: A progress report. *Br. J. Dis. Commun.* **16**, 159–174.

BAX, M. (1987). Paediatric assessment of the child with a speech and language disorder. In: *Language Development and Disorders,* W. Yule and M. Rutter (Eds). Oxford: SIMP, Blackwell Scientific and Lippincott.

BAX, M., HART, H. and JENKINS, S. (1980). Assessment of speech and language development in the young child. *Pediatrics* **66**, 350–354.

BEITCHAM, J.H., NAIR, R., CLEGG, M. and PATEL, P.G. (1986). Prevalence of speech and language disorders in five-year-old kindergarten children in the Ottowa-Carleton region. *J. Speech Hear. Dis.* **51**, 98–119.

BENTON, A. (1978). The cognitive functioning of children with developmental dysphasia. In: *Developmental Dysphasia,* M. Wyke (Ed.). London: Academic Press.

BERGER, M. (1987). What is a language disorder? *Proceedings of First International Symposium Specific Speech and Language Disorders in Children,* University of Reading. London: AFASIC.

BERNSTEIN, N. (1967). *The Coordination and Regulation of Movements.* Oxford: Pergamon.

BERRY, M.F. (1969). *Language Disorders of Children.* New York: Appleton-Century-Crofts.

BERRY, M.F. (1980). *Teaching Linguistically Handicapped Children.* Englewood Cliffs, New Jersey: Prentice-Hall.

BEVERIDGE, M. and CONTI-RAMSDEN, G. (1987). *Children with Language Disabilities.* Milton   Keynes: Open University Press.

BISHOP, D.V.M. (1979). Comprehension in developmental language disorders. *Dev. Med. Child Neurol* **21**, 225–238.

BISHOP, D.V.M. (1983). Comprehension of English syntax by profoundly deaf children. *J. Child Psychol. Psychiatr.* **24**, 415–434.

BISHOP, D.V.M. (1986). Some new data using the EPVT (full range version with a British sample) *Br. J. Dis. Commun.* **21**, 209–221.

BISHOP, D.V.M. (1987a). The causes of specific developmental language disorder (developmental dysphasia). *J. Child Psychol. Psychiat.* **28**, 1–8.

BISHOP, D.V.M. (1987b). The concept of comprehension in language disorders. *Proceedings of First International Symposium Specific Speech and Language Disorders in Children*, University of Reading. London: AFASIC.

BISHOP, D.V.M. (1989). Autism, Asperger's syndrome and semantic–pragmatic disorder: where are the boundaries? *Br. J. Dis. Commun.* **24**, 107–121.

BISHOP, D.V.M. and EDMUNDSON, A. (1986). Is otitis media a major cause of developmental language disorders? *Br. J. Dis. Commun.* **21**, 321–338.

BISHOP, D.V.M. and EDMUNDSON, A. (1987a). Language-impaired 4-year-olds. Distinguishing transient from persistent impairment. *J. Speech Hear. Dis.* **52**, 156–173.

BISHOP, D.V.M. and EDMUNDSON, A. (1987b). Specific language impairment as a maturational lag: evidence from longitudinal data on language and motor development. *Dev. Med. Child Neurol.* **29**, 442–449.

BISHOP, D.V.M. and ROSENBLOOM, L. (1987). Childhood language disorders. Classification and overview. In: *Language Development and Disorders*, W. Yule and M. Rutter (Eds). *Clinics in Developmental Medicine*. Oxford: SIMP, Blackwell Scientific and Lippincott.

BLAU, A., LAHEY, M. and OLEKSIUK-VELEZ, A. (1984). Planning goals for intervention. Can a language test serve as an alternative to a language sample? *J. Child Commun. Dis.* **72**, 27–37.

BLOOM, L. (1970). *Language Development. Form and Function in Developing Grammars.* Cambridge, Mass: MIT Press.

BLOOM, L. (1973). *One Word at a Time. The Use of Single-word Utterances before Syntax.* The Hague: Mouton.

BLOOM, L. and LAHEY, M. (1978). *Language Development and Language Disorders.* New York: J. Wiley.

BOOMER, D.S. and LAVER, J. (1968). Slips of the tongue. *Br. J. Dis. Commun.* **3**, 2–12.

BOUCHER, J. (1976). Is autism a language disorder? *Br. J. Dis. Commun.* **11**, 135–143.

BROADBENT, D. (1958). *Perception and Communication.* Oxford: Pergamon.

BROWN, A. (1975). The development of memory. In: *Advances in Child Development and Behavior 10*, H. Reese (Ed). New York: Academic Press.

BROWN, R. (1973). *A First Language. The Early Stages.* Cambridge, Mass: Harvard University Press.

BROWN, R. and BERKO, J. (1960). Word association and the acquisition of grammar. *Child Dev.* **31**, 1–14.

BROWNING, E. (1987). *I Can't See What You Are Saying.* London: Angel Press.

BRUNER, J. (1964). The course of cognitive growth. *Am. Psychol.* **19**, 1–15.

BRUNER, J. (1975). The ontogenesis of speech Acts. *J. Child Lang.* **2**, 1–15.

BRUNER, J. (1983a). *Child's Talk* New York: W.W. Norton.

BRUNER, J. (1983b). *In Search of Mind.* New York: Harper & Row.

BRYANT, P. (1985). The question of prevention. In: *Children's Written Language Difficulties*, M. Snowling (Ed.). Windsor: NFER Nelson.

BUTLER, D. (1987). *Cushla and her Books.* Harmondsworth: Penguin.

BUTLER, D. (1988). *Babies need Books.* Harmondsworth: Penguin.

BUTLER, K.G. (1984). Language processing. Half way up the down staircase. In: *Language Learning Disabilities in School Age Children*, G.P. Wallach and K.G. Butler (Eds). Baltimore: Williams & Wilkins.

(BYERS) BROWN, B. (1971a). *Speak for yourself.* Reading: Educational Explorers

BYERS BROWN, B. (1971b). A suggested rationale for the treatment of developmental disorders of language. In: *Applications of Linguistics*, G.E. Perrin and J.L. Trim (Eds). Selected papers of the Second International Conference of Applied Linguistics, Cambridge.

BYERS BROWN, B. (1976). Language vulnerability, speech delay and therapeutic intervention. *Br. J. Dis. Commun.* **11**, 43–56.

BYERS BROWN, B. (1981). *Speech Therapy: Principles and Practice.* Edinburgh: Churchill Livingstone.

BYERS BROWN, B. (1982). Clinical factors in language disorder: Core implicit and crisis induced. Paper presented at Annual Convention of American Speech, Language and Hearing Association, Toronto, Canada.

BYERS BROWN, B. (1985). Evidence upon which to act: The identification of communication disorders. *Jansson Memorial Lecture London. Br. J. Dis. Commun.* **20**, 3–18.

BYERS BROWN, B. (1987). Early identification of language disorders. *Proceedings of First International Symposium Specific Speech and Language Disorders in Children*, University of Reading. London: AFASIC.

BYERS BROWN, B. (1988). The utterances of one-year-old infants. *Proceedings of Child Language Conference*, University of Warwick (in press).

BYERS BROWN, B. and BEVERIDGE, M. (1979). *Language Disorders in Children*, Monograph, No. 1. London: College of Speech Therapists.

BYERS BROWN, B. and LEWIS, M. (1984). Speech–sound behaviour at one year of age. *Proceedings of Symposium on Research in Child Language Disorders*, University of Wisconsin, Madison, pp. 199–214.

BYERS BROWN, B., BENDERSKY, M. and CHAPMAN, T. (1986). The early utterances of preterm infants. *Br. J. Dis. Commun.* **21**, 307–320.

CAMARATA, A.S. and SCHWARTZ, R. (1985). Production of object words and action words: evidence for a relationship between phonology and semantics. *J. Speech Hear. Res.* **28**, 323–330.

CAMPBELL, R.N. (1979). Cognitive development and child language. In: *Language Acquisition*, P. Fletcher and M. Garman (Eds). Cambridge: Cambridge University Press.

CAPUTE, A.J., PALMER, F.B., SHAPIRO, B.K., WACHTEL, R.G., SCHMIDT, S. and ROSS, A. (1986). Clinical and auditory milestone scale: Prediction of cognition in infancy. *Dev. Med. Child Neurol.* **28**, 762–771.

CARAMAZZA, A. and ZURIF, E.B. (1978). Comprehension of center embedded sentences in aphasia and in development. In: *The Development and Breakdown of Language Functions: Parallels and Divergencies* Baltimore: The Johns Hopkins Press.

CHIAT, S. and HIRSON, A. (1987). From conceptual intention to utterances: a study of impaired language output in a child with developmental dysphasia. *Br. J. Dis. Commun.* **22**, 37–64.

COLLEGE OF SPEECH THERAPISTS (1988a). Position paper: The role of speech therapists in child language disability. College of Speech Therapists, London.

COLLEGE OF SPEECH THERAPISTS (1988b). Position paper 2/88: Education Act 1981, Guidelines for Speech Therapists. College of Speech Therapists, London.

COLLEGE OF SPEECH THERAPISTS (1989). City of Birmingham Polytechnic. School of Speech Therapy and University of Birmingham. College of Speech Therapists, London.

COLTHEART, M. (1987). Producing language. In: *Language Processing in Children and Adults*, M. Harris and M. Coltheart (Eds). London: Routledge, Keegan & Paul.

CONTI-RAMSDEN, G. (1987). Mother–child talk with language-impaired children *Proceedings of First International Symposium Specific Speech and Language Disorders in Children*, University of Reading. London: AFASIC.

CONTI-RAMSDEN, G. and GUNN, C. (1986). The development of conversational disability: a case study. *Br. J. Dis. Commun.* **21**, 339–351.

COOPER, J.M. (1985). Children with specific learning difficulties: the role of the speech therapist. In: *Children's Written Language Difficulties*, M. Snowling (Ed.). Windsor: NFER Nelson.

COOPER, J.M. and GRIFFITHS, C.P.S. (1978). Treatment and prognosis in developmental dysphasia. In: *Developmental Dysphasia*, M. Wyke (Ed.). London: Academic Press.

COOPER, J.M., MOODLEY, M. and REYNELL, J. (1978). *Helping Language Development.* London: Edward Arnold.

COPLAN J. (1983). *Early Language Milestone Scale.* Tulsa: Modern Education Corp.

COUPE, J. and GOLDBART, J. (1987). *Communication before Speech: Normal Development and Impaired Communication.* London: Croom Helm.

COYLE, J. (1983). Neurotransmitter systems in psychotic and cognitive behavior. Paper presented to the Symposium on Developmental Disabilities V. Autism and Related Disorders of Communication. Johns Hopkins Medical Center, Baltimore.

CRAIG, F. and TULVING, E. (1975). Depth of processing and retention of words in episodic memory. *J. Exp. Psychol. General* **104**, 268–294.

CRARY, M.A. (1984). A neurolinguistic perspective of developmental dyspraxia. *Commun. Dis.* **9**, 3.

CROMER, R.F. (1974). The development of language and cognition: the cognition hypothesis. In: *New Perspectives in Child Development*, B. Foss (Ed.). Harmondsworth: Penguin.

CROMER, R.F. (1978). The basis of childhood dysphasia: a linguistic approach. In: *Developmental Dysphasia*, M. Wyke (Ed.). London: Academic Press.

CRYSTAL, D. (1980). *Introduction to Language Pathology.* London: Edward Arnold.

CRYSTAL, D. (1981). *Clinical Linguistics. Disorders of communication.* Vienna: Springer-Verlag.

CRYSTAL, D. (1982a). Terms, time and teeth. *Br. J. Dis. Commun.* **17**, 3–19.

CRYSTAL, D. (1982b). *Profiling Linguistic Disability.* London: Edward Arnold.

CRYSTAL, D. (1986). *Listen to your Child.* Harmondsworth: Penguin.

CRYSTAL, D. (1987). Towards a 'bucket' theory of language disability: taking account of interaction between linguistic levels. *Clin. Linguist. Phonet.* **1**, 2–7.

CRYSTAL, D., FLETCHER, P. and GARMAN, M. (1976). *The Grammatical Analysis of Language Disability.* London: Edward Arnold.

CURTISS, S. (1977). *Genie: A psycholinguistic study of a modern day 'wild child'.* London: Academic Press.

DAMICO, J.S. (1988). The lack of efficacy in language therapy. A case study. *Lang. Speech Hearing Services in Schools,* **19**, 41–50.

DARLEY, F.L. and SPRIESTERSBACH, D. (1978). *Diagnostic methods in Speech Pathology.* New York: Harper & Row.

DEAN, E. and HOWELL, J. (1986). Developing linguistic awareness: a theoretically based approach to phonological disorders. *Br. J. Dis. Commun.* **21**, 223–238.

D'SOUZA, S.W., MCCARTNEY, E., NOLAN, M. and TAYLOR, I.G. (1981). Hearing, speech and language in survivors of severe prenatal asphyxia. *Arch. Dis. Child.* **56**, 563–566.

DE VILLIERS, J.G. and DE VILLIERS, P.A. (1978). *Language Acquisition.* Cambridge, Mass: Harvard University Press.

DEL PRIORE, C., VALANCE, S. and DAY, R. (1987). Understanding the communication disordered child: a developmental and observational perspective. Paper presented at *First International Symposium: Specific Speech and Language Disorders in Children,* University of Reading.

DOBBING, J. (1972). Growth of the brain. In: *Science Journal. The Human Brain.* London: Paladin.

DOUGLASS, R.L. (1983). Defining and describing clinical accountability. *Semin. Speech Lang.* **4**, 107–118.

DUXBURY, C. (1986). Syntactic comprehension and developmental language disability. *Unpublished dissertation for MSc,* University of London Institute of Neurology.

ECCLES, J. (1973). *The Understanding of the Brain.* New York: McGraw Hill.

EDWARDS, J.R. (1979). *Language and Disadvantage.* London: Edward Arnold.

EDWARDS, M. (1973). Developmental verbal apraxia. *Br. J. Dis. Commun.* **8**, 64–70.

EDWARDS, M. (1981). Assessment and remediation of speech. In: *Advances in the Management of Cleft Palate*, M. Edwards and A.C.H. Watson (Eds). Edinburgh: Churchill Livingstone.

EDWARDS, M. (1982). Verbal dyspraxia: a disorder of rhythm and seriation. *Unpublished pilot study.*

EDWARDS, M. (1984). *Disorders of Articulation: Aspects of Dysarthria and Dyspraxia. Disorders of Communication.* Vienna. Springer-Verlag.

EDWARDS, M. (1985). Terminology. Good descriptions are needed for clear diagnosis. *Speech Ther. Pract.* **1**, 20–21.

EDWARDS, M., BROWN, D., CAPE, J. and FOREMAN, D. (1984). Criteria for selection of children for speech therapy. *Unpublished report.* Funded by Department of Health and Social Services.

EISENSON, J. (1968). Developmental aphasia: a speculative view with therapeutic implications. *J. Speech Hear. Dis.* **33**, 3–13.

EISENSON, J. (1972). *Aphasia in Children.* New York: Harper & Row.

EISENSON, J. (1985). Central auditory disorders and developmental aphasia. Is there a difference? *Human Commun. (Canada)* **9**, 13–16.

EISENSON, J. (1986). Developmental (congenital) aphasia and acquired aphasia and dysphasia. *Human Commun. (Canada)* **10**, 5–9.

ELLIS ROBINSON, M.R. (1987). Provision and management for primary speech and language disorders in Australia. *Proceedings of First International Symposium: Specific speech and language disorders in children*, University of Reading. London: AFASIC.

FAIRBANKS, G. (1954). Systematic research in experimental phonetics. A theory of the speech mechanism as a servo mechanism. *J. Speech Hear. Dis.* **19**, 133–139.

FAUCETT, G.F. and CLIBBONS, J.S. (1983). The acquisition of signs by the mentally handicapped. *Br. J. Dis. Commun.* **18**, 13–21.

FEY, M.E. (1986). *Language Intervention with Young Children.* San Diego: College Hill Press.

FLETCHER, P. (1987). The basis of language impairment in children: a comment on Chiat and Hirson. *Br. J. Dis. Commun.* **22**, 65–72.

FLETCHER, P. and GARMAN, M. (1986). *The standardisation of an expressive language assessment procedure.* Department of Linguistic Sciences, University of Reading.

FRANKENBURG, W.K., FANDAL, A.W., SCIARELTO, W. and BURGESS, D. (1981). The newly abbreviated and revised Denver Developmental Screening Test. *J. Pediatr.* **33**, 335–399.

FROMKIN, V.A. (1968). Speculations of performance models. *J. Linguist.* **4**, 47–68.

FUNDUDIS, T., KOLVIN, I. and GARSIDE, R. (1979). *Speech Retarded and Deaf Children.* London: Academic Press.

FURROW, D. and NELSON, K. (1986). Another look at the motherese hypothesis: a reply to Gleitman. *J. Child Lang.* **13**, 153–167.

GALLAGHER, T.M. (1983). Pre assessment. A procedure for accommodating language use variability. In: *Pragmatic Assessment and Intervention*, T.M. Gallagher and C.A. Prutting (Eds). San Diego: College Hill Press.

GARRETT, M.F. (1980). Levels of processing in sentence production. In: *Language Production Vol. 1*, B. Butterworth (Ed.). London: Academic Press.

GARVEY, C. and KRAMER, T.L. (1988). The language of social pretend play. *Unpublished paper.*

GARVEY, M. and MUTTON, D.E. (1973). Sex chromosome aberrations and speech development. *Arch Dis. Child.* **48**, 937–941.

GATHERCOLE, S.E. and BADDELEY, A.D. (1989). Development of vocabulary in children depends upon short term phonological memory. *J. Memory Lang.* **28**, 200–213.

GERMAN, D.J. (1985). The use of specific semantic word categories in the diagnosis of dysnomic learning-disabled children. *Br. J. Dis Commun.* **20**, 143–154.

GERMAN, D.J. (1987). Spontaneous language profiles of children with word finding problems. *Lang. Speech Hear. Services in Schools* **18**, 206–216.

GESCHWIND, N. and LEVITSKY, W. (1968). Human Brain: Left–right asymmetries in temporal speech region. *Science* **161**, 186–187.

GIBSON, D. and INGRAM, D. (1983). The onset of comprehension in a language delayed child. *Appl. Psycholinguist.* **4**, 359–370.

GLEITMAN, L., NEWPORT, C. and GLEITMAN, H. (1984). The current status of the motherese hypothesis. *J. Child Lang.* **11**, 43–79.

GOLINKOFF, R.M. (1983). The preverbal negotiation of failed messages: insights into the transition period. In: *The Transition from Prelinguistic to Linguistic Communication*, R.M. Golinkoff (Ed.). Hillsdale, NJ: Lawrence Erlbaum.

GOODMAN, R. (1987). The developmental neurobiology of language. In: *Language Development and Disorders*, W. Yule and M. Rutter (Eds). Oxford: SIMP, Blackwell Scientific and Lippincott.

GORDON, N. (1966). The child who does not talk. Problems of diagnosis with special reference to children with severe auditory agnosia. *Br. J. Dis. Commun.* **1**, 78–84.

GORDON, N. (1987). Developmental disorders of language. In: *Language Development and Disorders*, W. Yule and M. Rutter (Eds). Oxford: SIMP, Blackwell Scientific and Lippincott.

GORDON, N. and MCKINLAY, I. (1980). *Helping Clumsy Children.* Edinburgh: Churchill Livingstone.

GREENE, M.C.L. (1963). A comparison of children with delayed speech due to coordination disorder or language learning difficulty. *Speech Pathol. Ther.* **6**, 69–77.

GREENE, M.C.L. (1964). Differential diagnosis of developmental aphasia. *Speech Pathol. Ther.* **7**, 84–93.

GREENE, M.C.L. (1967). Speechless and backward at three. *Br. J. Dis. Commun.* **2**, 134–145.

GRIFFITHS, C.P.S. (1964). Treatment of developmental aphasia. *Speech Pathol. Ther.* **7**, 95–99.

GRIFFITHS, C.P.S. (1969). A follow up study of children with disorders of speech. *Br. J. Dis. Commun.* **4**, 46–56.

GRIFFITHS, C.P.S. (1972). *Developmental Aphasia: An Introduction.* London: ICAA (now ICAN).

GRUNWELL, P. (1975). The phonological analysis of language disorders. *Br. J. Dis. Commun.* **10**, 1–31.

GRUNWELL, P. (1980a). Developmental language disorders at the phonological level. In: *Language Disabilities in Children*, M. Jones (Ed.). Lancaster: MTP Press.

GRUNWELL, P. (1980b). Procedures for child assessment: a review. *Br. J. Dis. Commun.* **15**, 189–203.

GRUNWELL, P. (1981). *The Nature of Phonological Disability in Children.* London: Academic Press.

GRUNWELL, P. (1982a). *Clinical Phonology.* London: Croom Helm.

GRUNWELL, P. (1982b). Review of natural process analysis: L.D. Shriberg and J. Kwiatkowski. *Br. J. Dis. Commun.* **17**, 155–156.

GRUNWELL, P. and RUSSELL, J. (1987). Vocalisations before, and after cleft palate surgery: a pilot study. *Br. J. Dis. Commun.* **22**, 1–18.

GUBBAY, S.S. (1975). *The Clumsy Child.* Philadelphia: WB Saunders.

GURALNICK, M.J. and BENNETT, F.C. (Eds). (1987). The framework for early intervention. In: *The Effectiveness of Early Intervention for At-risk and Handicapped Children.* New York: Academic Press.

HABER, R.N. and STANDING, L.G. (1969). Direct measures of long term visual storage. *Q. J. Exp. Psychol.* **21**, 43–54.

HALL, P.K. and TOMBLIN, J.B. (1978). A follow-up of children with articulation and language disorders. *J. Speech Hear. Dis.* **43**, 227–241.

HALLIDAY, M.A.K. (1963). The tones of English. *Arch. Linguist.* **15**, 1–28.

HALLIDAY, M.A.K. (1975). *Learning how to Mean. Explorations in the development of language.* London: Edward Arnold.

HAMILTON, P. and OWRID, H.L. (1974). Comparison of hearing impairment and socio-cultural disadvantage in relation to verbal retardation. *Br. J. Audiol.* **8**, 27–32.

HARRIS, J. (1984). Teaching children to develop language: the impossible dream. In: *Remediating Children's Language: Behavioural and Naturalistic Approaches*, D. Müller (Ed.). London: Croom Helm.

HASENSTAB, S.M. (1987). *Language Learning and Otitis Media.* London: Taylor & Francis.

HAYNES, C. (1986). Assessment for identification and for therapy. In: *Advances in Working with Language-disordered Children.* Invalid Children's Aid Association Nationwide (ICAN), Conference Proceedings, London.

HEALTH FOR ALL CHILDREN (1989). *Report of Joint Working Party Preschool Child Surveillance.* Oxford: Medical Publications.

HEBB, D.O. (1972). *Textbook of Psychology*, 3rd edn. Philadelphia: WB Saunders.

HERBERT, G. and WEDELL, K. (1970). Communication handicaps of children with specific language deficiency. Paper presented at Annual Conference of British Psychological Society, Southampton.

HEYWOOD, C.A. and CANAVAN, A.G.M. (1987). Developmental neuropsychological correlates of language. In: *Language Development and Disorders*, W. Yule and M. Rutter (Eds). Oxford: SIMP, Blackwell Scientific and Lippincott.

HILL, A., HOWELL, J. and WATERS, D. (1988). A research study of therapeutic intervention. *Proceedings of the Child Language Conference*, University of Warwick, in press.

HITCH, G.J. and HALLIDAY, M.S. (1983). Working memory in children. *Phil. Trans. R. Soc. B* **302**, 325–340.

HOWELL, J. and DEAN, E. (1987). I think that's a noisy sound: reflection and learning in the therapeutic situation. *Child Lang. Teach. Ther.* **3**, 259–266.

HOWELL, J. and MCCARTNEY, E. (1989). Approaches to remediation. In: *Developmental Speech Disorders. Current Issues and Implications*, P. Grunwell (Ed.). Edinburgh: Churchill Livingstone.

HUBBELL, R.D. (1981). *Children's Language Disorders.* Englewood Cliffs, NJ: Prentice-Hall.

HUTT, E. (1986). *Teaching Language-disordered Children: A Structured Curriculum.* London: Edward Arnold.

HUTT, E. and DONLAN, C. (1987). *Adequate Provision? A survey of language units.* Invalid Children's Aid Association Nationwide (ICAN), 198 City Road, London EC1V 2PH.

ICAN (1988). *Units for Primary School Children with Speech and Language Disorders. Suggested Guidelines.*

INGRAM, D. (1974). Phonological rules in young children. *J. Child. Lang.* **1**, 49–64.

INGRAM, D. (1976). *Phonological Disability in Children.* London: Edward Arnold.

INGRAM, D. (1981). *Procedures for the Phonological Analysis of Children's Speech*, Baltimore: University Park Press.

INGRAM, D. (1987). Categories of phonological disorder. *Proceedings of First International Symposium: Specific Speech and Language Disorders in Children*, University of Reading. London: AFASIC.

INGRAM, T.T.S. (1959). Specific developmental disorders of speech in childhood. *Brain* **82**, 450–467.

INGRAM, T.T.S. (1965). Specific retardation of speech development. *Speech Pathol. Ther* **8**, 3–11.

ISRAEL, L. (1984). Word knowledge and word retrieval. Phonological and semantic strategies. In: *Language Learning Disabilities in School-age Children*, G.P. Wallach and K.G. Butler (Eds). Baltimore: Williams & Wilkins.

JACOBSON, R. (1968). *Child Language, Aphasia and Phonological Universals.* The Hague: Mouton.

JERGER, S., JERGER, J., ALFORD, B.R. and ABRAMS, S. (1983). Development of speech intelligibility in children with recurrent otitis media. *Ear Hear.* 4, 138–145.

JOHNSON, J.R. and SCHERY, T.K. (1976). The use of grammatical morphemes by children with communication disorders. In: *Normal and Deficient Child Language*, D.M. Morehead and A.E. Morehead (Eds). Baltimore: University Park Press.

KAGAN, J. (1971). *Change and Continuity in Infancy.* New York: J Wiley.

KAGAN, J. (1988). Paediatric diagnosis of language delay. *Pediatrics* in press.

KAHMI, A. (1985). Questioning the value of large numerical multivariate studies: a response to Schery. *J. Speech Hear. Dis.* 50, 288–290.

KELLETT, B., LEE, B. and MOBLEY, P. (1984). The Kellett Colour Coding Scheme. Private publication, Central Manchester Health Authority.

KELLY, D.J. and RICE, M.L. (1986). A strategy for language assessment of young children: a combibation of two approaches. *Lang. Speech Hear. Services in Schools* 17, 83–94.

KELSO, J.A. SCOTT (Ed.) (1982). Concepts and issues in motor behavior. In: *Human Motor Behavior.* Hillsdale NJ: Lawrence Erlbaum.

KENT, R.D. (1984). Psychobiology of speech development: co-emergence of language and a movement system. *Am. J. Physiol.* 246, 855–942.

KING, R.R., JONES, C. and LASKY, E. (1982). In retrospect: a fifteen year follow-up report of speech and language-disordered children. *Lang. Speech Hear. Services in Schools* 13, 24–32.

KIRK, U. (Ed.) (1983). Toward an understanding of the neuropsychology of language, reading and spelling. *Neuropsychology of Language Reading and Spelling.* London: Academic Press.

KOZHEVNIKOV, V.A. and CHISTOVICH, L.A. (1965). *Speech Articulation and Perception.* Moscow: Nauka. (Trans. US Dept of Commerce. Joint Publications Service, Washington DC.)

LARGO, R.H. and HOWARD, J.A. (1979). Developmental progression in play behaviour of children between nine and thirty months: 2. Spontaneous play and language development. *Dev. Med. Child Neurol.* 21, 492–503.

LASHLEY, K.S. (1951). The problem of serial order in behaviour. In: *Cerebral Mechanisms and Behavior*, L.A. Jeffress (Ed.). New York: J. Wiley.

LAVER, J. (1977). Neurolinguistic aspects of speech production. In: *Grundebegriffe und Haupströmungen der Linguistisk*, C. Gutnecht (Ed.). Hamburg: Hoffman und Campe.

LEA, J. (1965). A language scheme for children suffering from receptive aphasia. *Speech Pathol. Ther.* 8, 58–68.

LEA, J. (1980). The association between rhythmic ability and language ability. In: *Language Disability in Children*, F.M. Jones (Ed.). Lancaster: MTP Press.

LEA, J. (1986). A follow-up study of severely speech and language handicapped school leavers. Paper presented at ICAN Conference Advances in Working with Language-disordered Children, London.

LENNEBERG, E. (1967). *Biological foundation of language.* New York: J. Wiley

LEONARD, L. (1972). What is deviant language? *J. Speech Hear. Dis.* 37, 427–446.

LEONARD, L. (1981). Facilitating language skills in children with specific language impairment. *Appl. Psycholinguist.* 2, 89–118.

LEONARD, L., PRUTTING, C., PEROZZI, J. and BERKEY, R.K. (1978). Non standardised approach to the assessment of language behavior. *ASHA* 20, 371–379.

LETTS, C. (1985). Linguistic interaction in Clinic: How do therapists do therapy? *Child Lang. Teach. Ther.* 1, 321–331.

LEVITT, L. and MUIR, J. (1983). Which three-year-olds need speech therapy? Use of Levitt–Muir Screening Test. *Health Visitor* 56, 454–456.

LEWIS, M. (1977). Social behaviour and language acquisition. In: *Interaction, Communication and the Development of Language*, M. Lewis and L.A. Rosenbloom (Eds). New York: J. Wiley.

LEWIS, M. and BENDERSKY, M. (1989). Cognitive and motor differences among low birth-weight infants: Impact of intraventricular haemorrhage, medical risk and social class. *Pediatrics* **83**, 187–192.

LEWIS, M. and FREEDLE, R. (1973). Mother–infant dyad: The cradle of meaning. In: *Communication and Affect: Language and Thought*, P. Pliner, L. Kramer and T. Alloway (Eds). New York: Academic Press.

LEWIS, M., BYERS BROWN, B. and MICHALSON, L. (1984). Survey of professionals who assess young children for communication disorders. *Report from the Institute for the Study of Child Development.* Robert Wood Johnson Medical School, NJ.

LEWIS, M., BYERS BROWN, B., LANEY, M., MICHALSON, L., HADZIMICHALIS, D. and JASKIER, J. (1985). Screening and assessment. A systems approach to improving the identification and management of communication disorders in young children. Presentation to International Congress on the Education of the Deaf, Manchester.

LIBERMAN, A.M., COOPER, F.S., HARRIS, K.S., MACNEILAGE, P.F. and STUDDERT-KENNEDY, M. (1964). Some observations on a model of speech perception. In: *Models for the Perception of Speech and Visual Form.* Cambridge, Mass: MIT Press.

LIBERMAN, A.M., COOPER, F.S., SHANKWEILER, D.P. and STUDDERT-KENNEDY, M. (1967). Perception of the speech code. *Psychol. Rev.* **74**, 431–461.

LIEVEN, E.V.M. (1978). Conversations between mothers and young children: Individual differences and their possible implication for the study of language learning. In: *Development of Communication*, N. Waterson and C. Snow (Eds). New York: J. Wiley.

LIEVEN, E.V.M. (1982). Context, process and progress in young children's speech. In: *Children Thinking Through Language*, M. Beveridge (Ed.). London: Edward Arnold.

LINDSAY, G. (Ed.) (1984). *Screening for Children with Special Needs.* London: Croom Helm.

LLOYD, P. (1982). Talking to some purpose. In: *Children thinking through Language,* M. Beveridge (Ed.). London: Edward Arnold.

LOCKE, A. (1985). *Living Language.* Windsor: NFER.

LOCKE, A. (1989). Screening and intervention with children with speech and language difficulties in mainstream schools. In: *Child Language Disability: Implications in an Educational Setting*, K. Mogford and J. Sadler (Eds). Clevedon: Avon Multilingual Matters.

LOCKE, J.L. (1980). The inference of speech perception in the phonologically disordered child. Parts 1 & 2. *J. Speech Hear. Dis.* **45**, 431–468.

LOCKE, J.L. (1983). *Phonological Acquisition and Change.* New York: Academic Press.

LOCKE, J.L. (1986). The linguistic significance of language. In: *Precursors of Early Speech*, B. Lindblom and R. Zetterstrom (Eds). *Werner-Gren International Symposium Series, 44.* Basingstoke: MacMillan Press. (New York: Stockton Press.)

LUDLOW, C. and COOPER, J.A. (Eds) (1983). *Genetic Aspects of Speech and Language Disorders.* New York: Academic Press.

LUND, N.J. (1986). Family events and relationships. *Seminars in Speech and Language*, Vol. 4. New York: Thième Medical.

LUND, N. and DUCHAN, J. (1983, 1987). *Assessing Children's Language in Naturalistic Contexts*, 1st and 2nd edns. Englewood Cliffs, NJ: Prentice-Hall.

LURIA, A.R. (1970). *Traumatic Aphasia.* The Hague: Mouton.

LURIA, A.R. (1973). *The Working Brain.* London: Allen Lane, The Penguin press.

LURIA, A.R. (1976). *Basic Problems of Neurolinguistics.* The Hague: Mouton.

LYONS, J. (1977). *Semantics*, Vols 1 and 2. Cambridge: Cambridge University Press.

MCCARTHY, D. (1930). *The language Development of the Pre School Child.* Child Welfare Monographs. Series 4. Minneapolis: University of Minneapolis Press.

MCCAULEY, R.J. and SWISHER, L. (1984). Use and misuse of norm-referenced tests in clinical assessment: A hypothetical case. *J. Speech Hear. Dis.* **49**, 338–348.

MCGINNIS, M. (1963). *Aphasic Children*. Washington DC: Alexander Graham Bell Association for the Deaf Inc.

MCLAUGHLIN, C.S. and GULLOW, D.F. (1984). Comparison of three formal methods of preschool language assessment. *Lang. Speech Hear. Services in Schools* **15**, 145–153.

MCTEAR, M.F. (1985). Pragmatic disorders: a question of direction. *Br. J. Dis. Commun.* **20**, 119–127.

MacKEITH, R. and RUTTER, M. (1972). A note on the prevalence of speech and language disorders. In: *The Child with Delayed Speech*, M. Rutter and J.A.M. Martin (Eds). *Clinics in Developmental Medicine* 43. London: SIMP with Heineman Medical.

MacNAMARA, J. (1972). Cognitive basis of language learning in infants. *Psychol. Rev.* **77**, 1–13.

MacNEILAGE, P.F. (1970). Motor control and serial ordering of speech. *Psychol. Rev.* **75**, 182–196.

MARGE, M. (1972). The general problem of language disabilities in children. In: *The Principles of Childhood Language Disabilities*, J.V. Irwin and M. Marge (Eds). New York: Appleton-Century-Crofts.

MARGE, M. (1984). The prevention of communication disorders. *ASHA* **26**, 29–34.

MARSHALL, J.C. (1983). Preface to *Aphasiology*, A.H. Lecours, F.L'Hermitte and B. Bryans. London: Baillière Tindall.

MARSLEN-WILSON, W.D. and TYLER, L.K. (1980). The temporal structure of spoken language understanding. *Cognition* **8**, 1–71.

MASIDLOVER, M. and KNOWLES' W.(1982). *The Derbyshire Language Scheme*. Obtainable from the authors, Derbyshire Education Authority.

MENYUK, P. and LOONEY, P.L. (1972). Relationships among components of the grammar in language disorders. *J. Speech Hear. Res.* **15**, 395–406.

MENYUK, P., LIEBERGOTT, J. and SCHULTZ, M. (1986). Predicting phonological development. In: *Precursors of Early Speech*, B. Lindblom and R. Zetterstrom (Eds). *Werner-Gren International Symposium Series. 44.* Basingstoke: Macmillan Press. (New York: Stockton Press.)

MILLER, G.A. (1967). The magical number of 7 plus or minus 2. *The Psychology of Communication*. Harmondsworth: Penguin.

MILLER, J.F. (1978). Assessing children's language behavior: A developmental process approach. In: *Bases of Language Intervention*, R.L. Schiefelbusch (Ed.). Baltimore: University Park Press.

MILLER, J.F. (1981). *Assessing Language Production in Children*. London: Edward Arnold.

MILLER, J.F. (1987). A grammatical characterization of language disorder. In: *Proceedings of First International Symposium: Specific Speech and Language Disorders in Children*, University of Reading. London: AFASIC.

MILLER, J.F., YODER, D.E. and SCHIEFELBUSCH, R. (Eds) (1983). *Contemporary Issues in Language Intervention*. Rockville, MD: ASHLA.

MILLER, L. (1984). Problem solving and language remediation. In: *Language Learning Disabilities in School Aged Children,* G.P. Wallach and K.G. Butler (Eds). Baltimore: Williams and Wilkins.

MORAY, N. (1972). *Listening and Attention*. Harmondsworth, Middlesex: Penguin Books.

MORGAN-BARRY, R.A. (1988). Language use versus phonology versus prosody: A spin-off effect. *Unpublished paper.*

MORLEY, M.E. (1960). Developmental receptive–expressive dysphasia. *Speech Pathol. Ther.* **3**, 64–76.

MORLEY, M.E. (1972). *Development and Disorders of Speech in Childhood*, 3rd edn. Edinburgh: Churchill Livingstone.

MORLEY, M.E. (1973). Receptive/expressive developmental aphasia. *Br. J. Dis. Commun.* **8**, 47–53.

MORLEY, M., COURT, S.D.M. and MILLER, H. (1954). *Br. Med. J.* **1**, 8.

MORTON, J. (1978). Facilitation in word recognition: experiments causing change in the logogen model. In: *Proceedings of the Conference on the Processing of Visible Language*, P.A. Kolers, M.E. Wrolstad and H. Bouma (Eds). New York: Plenum.

MOUNTCASTLE, V.B. (Ed.) (1980). *Medical Physiology*, 14th edn. St Louis: C.V. Mosby.

MOWRER, O.M. (1952). Speech development in the young child. 1. The autism theory of speech development and some clinical applications. *J. Speech Hear. Dis.* **17**, 260–268.

MÜLLER, D.J., MUNRO, S. and CODE, C. (1981). *Language Assessment for Remediation*. London: Croom Helm.

MUMA, J.R. (1978). *Language Handbook. Concepts, Assessment, Intervention*. Englewood Cliffs, NJ: Prentice-Hall.

MUMA, J.R. (1983). Speech–language pathology: Emerging clinical expertise in language. In: *Pragmatic Assessment and Intervention in Language*, T.M. Gallagher and C.A. Prutting (Eds). San Diego: College Hill Press.

MYSACK, E.D. (1976). *Pathologies of Speech Systems*. Baltimore, MD: Williams & Wilkins.

NATION, J. and ARAM, D. (1977). *Diagnosis of Speech and Language Disorders*. St Louis: C.V. Mosby.

NETSELL, R. (1986). The acquisition of speech motor control. In: *A Neurobiologic View of Speech Production and the Dysarthrias*. San Diego: College Hill Press.

NOLAN, C. (1987). *Under the Eye of the Clock*. London: Weidenfeld & Nicholson.

OLLER, D.K. (1980). The emergence of the sounds of speech in infancy. In: *Child Phonology, Volume 1 Production*, G.H. Yeni-Komshian, J.F. Kavanagh and C.A. Ferguson (Eds). New York: Academic Press.

OWRID, H.L. (1970). Hearing impairment and verbal attainment in Primary School children. *Educ. Res.* **12**, 209–214.

PANAGOS, J.M. (1982). The case against the autonomy of phonological disorders in children. *Semin. Speech Lang. Hear.* **3**, 172–182.

PANAGOS, J.M. and BOBKOFF, K. (1984). Beliefs about developmental apraxia of speech. *Austr. J. Human Commun. Dis.* **12**, 40–53.

PANAGOS, J.M., QUINE, M.E. and KLICH, R.J. (1979). Syntactic and phonological influences on children's articulation. *J. Speech Hear. Res.* **22**, 829–840.

PANAGOS, J.M., BOBKOFF, K. and SCOTT, C.M. (1986). Discourse analysis of language intervention. *Child Lang. Teach. Ther.* **2**, 211–229.

PANAGOS, J.M., BOBKOFF-KATZ, K., KOVARSKY, D. and PRELOCK, P.A. (1988). The non-verbal component of clinical lessons. *Child Lang. Teach. Ther.* **4**, 228–296.

PARADISE, J.L. (1981). Otitis media in early life. How hazardous to development? A critical review of the evidence. *Pediatrics* **68**, 869–873.

PAUL, R. and COHEN, D.J. (1987). Outcomes of severe disorders of language acquisition. *J. Autism Dev. Dis.* **17**, 405–421.

PENFIELD, W. and ROBERTS, L. (1959). *Speech and Brain Mechanisms*. Princeton, NJ: Princeton University Press.

PETRIE, I. (1975). Characteristics and progress of a group of language disordered children with receptive difficulties. *Br. J. Dis. Commun.* **10**, 122–133.

PROCTOR, A. (1982). Use of linguistic input in clinical assessment. Miniseminar presented at Annual Convention of American Speech Language and Hearing Association, Toronto.

PRUTTING, C.A. and KIRCHNER, D.M. (1983). Applied pragmatics. In: *Pragmatic Assessment and Intervention: Issues in Language*, T.M. Gallagher and C.A. Prutting (Eds). San Diego: College Hill Press.

PRUTTING, C.A., GALLAGHER, T. and MULAC, A. (1975). The expressive portion of the NWSST compared to a spontaneous language sample. *J. Speech Hear. Dis.* **40**, 40–49.

PURPURA, D.P. and YAHR, M.D. (1966). *The Thalamus.* New York: Columbia University Press.

RANDALL, D., REYNELL, J. and CURWEN, M. (1974). A study of language development in a sample of three-year-old children *Br. J. Dis. Commun.* **9**, 3–16.

RAPIN, I. and ALLEN, D.A. (1983). Developmental language disorders: nosological considerations. In: *Neuropsychology of Language, Reading and Spelling*, U. Kirk (Ed.). New York: Academic Press.

RAPIN, I. and ALLEN, D.A. (1987). Developmental dysphasia and autism in pre-school children. In: *Proceedings of First International Symposium: Specific Speech and Language Disorders in Children*, University of Reading. London: AFASIC.

REES, N. (1973). Auditory processing factors in language disorders: the view from Procrustes' bed. *J. Speech Hear. Dis.* **38**, 304–315.

RESCORLA, L. (1984). Language delay in two-year-olds. Paper presented at Fourth International Symposium of Infant Studies, New York.

REYNELL, J.K. (1969). A developmental approach to language disorders. *Br. J. Dis. Commun.* **4**, 38–40.

RICE, M. (1983). Contemporary accounts of the cognition/language relationship. Implications for speech–language clinicians. *J. Speech Hear. Dis.* **48**, 347–359.

RIPICH, D.N. and PANAGOS, J.M. (1985). Accessing children's knowledge of sociolinguistic rules for speech therapy lessons. *J. Speech Hear. Dis.* **50**, 346–355.

RIPLEY, K. (1987). Counselling children with specific speech and language disorders. *Proceedings of First International Symposium Specific Speech and Language Disorders in Children*, University of Reading. London: AFASIC.

ROBINSON, R.J. (1987). The causes of language disorder. *Proceedings of First Internation al Symposium Specific Speech and Language Disorders in Children*, University of Reading. London: AFASIC.

ROSENBEK, J. (1974). Treatment of developmental apraxia of speech: A case study. *Lang. Speech Hear. Services in Schools* **5**, 13–22.

RUTTER, M. (Ed.) (1984). Issues and prospects in developmental neuropsychiatry. In: *Developmental Neuropsychiatry.* Edinburgh: Churchill Livingstone.

RUTTER, M. (1987). Developmental language disorders: Some thoughts on causes and correlates. *Proceedings of First International Symposium on Specific Speech and Language Disorders in Children*, University of Reading. London: AFASIC.

RUTTER, M. and LORD, C. (1987). Language disorder associated with psychiatric disturbance. In: *Language Development and Disorders*, W. Yule and M. Rutter (Eds). Oxford: SIMP, Blackwell Scientific and Lippincott.

RUTTER, M., BARTAK, L. and NEWMAN, S. (1971). Autism: A central disorder of cognition and language? In: *Infantile Autism. Concepts Characteristics and Treatment*, M. Rutter (Ed.). Edinburgh: Churchill Livingstone.

RUTTER, M., TIZARD, J. and WHITMORE, K. (1970). *Education Health and Behaviour.* London: Longmans.

SATZ, P. and ZAIDE, J. (1983). Sex differences: Clues or myths? In: *Genetic Aspects of Speech and Language Disorders*, C. Ludlow and J.A. Cooper (Eds). New York: Academic Press.

SAVIC, S. (1980). *How Twins Learn to Talk.* London: Academic Press.

SCHERY, T.K. (1985). Correlates of language development in language-disordered children. *J. Speech Hear. Dis.* **50**, 73–83.

SEMEL, E.M. and WIIG, E. (1980). *Clinical Evaluation of Language Functions.* Columbus, Ohio: Charles Merrill. (Also revised by E. Wiig, CELF, Psychological Corp.)

SHATTUCK-HUFFNAGEL, S. (1979). Speech errors as evidence for a serial-ordering mechanism in sentence production. In: *Sentence Processing: Psycholinguistic*

Studies presented to Merrill Garrett, W.H. Cooper and E.C.T. Walker (Eds). Hillsdale, NJ: Lawrence Erlbaum.

SHATZ, M. (1977). Relationship between cognitive processes and the development of communicative skills. In: *Nebraska Symposium on Motivation*. Lincoln, Nebraska: University of Nebraska.

SHERIDAN, M. (1973). Children of 7 with marked speech defects. *Br. J. Dis. Commun.* **8**, 9–16.

SHRIBERG, L.D. and KWIATKOWSKI, J. (1982). Phonological disorders 1: A diagnostic classification system. *J. Speech Hear. Dis.* **42**, 242–255.

SHRIBERG, L.D. and SMITH, A.J. (1983). Phonological correlates of middle ear involvement in speech-delayed children: a methodological note. *J. Speech Hear. Res.* **26**, 293–297.

SIEGEL, G.M. (1987). The limits of science in communication disorders. *J. Speech Hear. Dis.* **52**, 306–312.

SIEGEL, G.M., KATSUKI, J. and POTECHIN, G. (1985). Response to contemporary accounts of the cognition/language relationship. *J. Speech Hear. Dis.* **50**, 281–317.

SILVA, P.A. (1980). The prevalence, stability and significance of developmental language delay in pre-school children. *Dev. Med. Child Neurol.* **22**, 768–777.

SILVA, P.A. (1987). Epidemiology: Longitudinal course and some associated factors. In: *Language Development and Disorders*, W. Yule and M. Rutter (Eds). Oxford: SIMP, Blackwell Scientific and Lippincott.

SILVA, P.A. and FERGUSON, D. (1980). Some factors contributing to language development in three-year-old children. *Br. J. Dis. Commun.* **15**, 200–214.

SILVA, P.A., MCGEE, R.O. and WILLIAMS, S.M. (1983). Developmental language delay from three to seven years and its significance for low intelligence and reading difficulties at age seven. *Dev. Med. Child Neurol.* **25**, 783–793.

SINCLAIR DE ZWART, H. (1969). Developmental psycholinguistics. In: *Studies in Cognitive Development*, D. Elkind and J. Flavell (Eds). Oxford: Oxford University Press.

SKINNER, B.F. (1957). *Verbal Behavior.* New York: Appleton-Century-Crofts.

SMITH, N. (1973). *The Acquisition of Phonology: A case study.* Oxford: Oxford University Press.

SNOW, C.E. (1972). Mothers' speech to children learning language. *Child Dev.* **13**, 549–565.

SNOW, C.E. and FERGUSON, C.A. (Eds) (1977). *Talking to Children: Language Input and Acquisition.* Cambridge: Cambridge University Press.

SNOWLING, M. (Ed.) (1985a). Postscript: Some consistencies and contradictions: directions for future research. In: *Children's Written Language Difficulties*. Windsor: NFER.

SNOWLING, M. (1985b). Dyslexia care – the therapist's crucial role. *Speech Ther. Pract.* **13**, 21–22.

SNOWLING, M.J. (1987). The assessment of reading problems in specific language impairment. *Proceedings of First International Symposium: Specific Speech and Language Disorders in Children*, University of Reading. London: AFASIC.

SNYDER, L. (1982). Defining language-disordered children: Disordered or just 'Low Verbal' normal? *Proceedings of Third Symposium on Research in Child Language Disorders*, Madison, Wisconsin.

SNYDER-MCCLEAN, L. and MCCLEAN, J.E. (1987). Effectiveness of early intervention for children with language and communicative disorders. In: *The Effectiveness of Early Intervention for At-risk and Handicapped Children*, M.J. Guralnick and F.C. Bennett (Eds). New York: Academic Press.

SONKSEN, P. (1979). The neurodevelopmental and paediatric findings associated with significant disabilities of language development. *Unpublished MD Thesis*, University of London.

SPENCE, J.C., WALTON, W.S., MILLER, F.J.W. and COURT, S.D.M. (1954). *A Thousand Families in Newcastle upon Tyne.* Durham: Durham University Press.

STACKHOUSE, J. (1982). An investigation of reading and spelling performance in speech-disordered children. *Br. J. Dis. Commun.* **17**, 53–60.

STACKHOUSE, J. (1985). Segmentation speech and spelling difficulties. In: *Children's Written Language Difficulties*, M. Snowling (Ed.). Windsor: NFER.

STARK, R.E. (1981). Stages of speech development in the first year of life. In: *Child Phonology, Volume 1 Production*, G.H. Yeni-Komshian, J.F. Kavanagh and C.A. Ferguson (Eds). New York: Academic Press.

STARK, R.E. and TALLAL, P. (1981). Selection of children with specific language impairment. *J. Speech Hear. Dis.* **46**, 114–122.

STARK, R.E., MELLITS, E. and TALLAL, P. (1983). Behavioral attributes of speech and language disorders. In: *Genetic Aspects of Speech and Language Disorders*, C.L. Ludlow and J.A. Cooper (Eds). New York: Academic Press.

STARK, R.E., TALLAL, P. and MELLITS, E. (1985). Expressive language and perceptual motor abilities in language-impaired children. *Human Commun. (Canada)* **9**, 23–28.

STARK, R.E., BERNSTEIN, L.E., CONDINO, R., BENDER, M., TALLAL, P. and CATTS, H. (1984). Four year follow-up study of language-impaired children. *Ann. Dyslexia* **34**, 49–68.

STELMACH, G.E. (1982). Information-processing framework for understanding human motor behavior. In: *Human Motor Behavior*, J. Scott Kelso (Ed.). Hillsdale, NJ: Lawrence Erlbaum.

STELMACH, G.E., KELSO, J.A.S. and WALLACE, S.A. (1975). Preselection in short term motor memory. *J. Exp. Psychol.* **1**, 745–755.

STEVENSON, J. and RICHMAN, N. (1976). The prevalence of language delay in a population of three-year-old children and its association with general retardation. *Dev. Med. Child Neurol.* **18**, 431–441.

STEVENSON, P., BAX, M. and STEVENSON, J. (1982). The evaluation of home-based speech therapy for language delayed pre-school children in an inner city area. *Br. J. Dis. Commun.* **17**, 141–148.

STROMINGER, A.Z. and BASHIR, A.S. (1977). A nine year follow-up of language-delayed children. Paper presented at Annual Convention of the American Speech Language and Hearing Association, Chicago.

TALLAL, P. (1987). The neuropsychology of developmental language disorders *Proceedings of First International Symposium: Specific Speech and Language Disorders in Children*, University of Reading. London: AFASIC.

TALLAL, P. and PIERCY, M. (1978). Defects of auditory perception in children with developmental dysphasia. In: *Developmental Dysphasia*, M. Wyke (Ed.). London: Academic Press.

TAYLOR, I.G. (1964). *Neurological Mechanisms of Speech and Hearing in Children.* Manchester: Manchester University Press.

TAYLOR, I.G. (1966). Hearing in relation to language disorders in children. *Br. J. Dis. Commun.* **1**, 11–20.

TAYLOR, O.L. (1982). Language differences. In: *Human Communication Disorders*, G.H. Shames and E.H. Wiig (Eds). Columbus, Ohio: Charles Merrill.

TEELE, D.W., KLEIN, J.O. ROSNER, B.A. and THE GREATER BOSTON OTITIS MEDIA STUDY GROUP (1984). Otitis media with effusion during the first three years of life, and development of language. *Pediatrics* **74**, 282–287.

TEW, B. (1979). The 'Cocktail Party Syndrome' in children with hydrocephalus and spina bifida. *Br. J. Dis Commun.* **14**, 89–101.

THAL, O, and BATES, E. (1988). Language and gesture in late talkers. *J. Speech Hear. Res.* **31**, 115–123.

THOMAS, M.E. (1969). Assessment and treatment of receptive and executive aphasia in identical twin boys. *Br. J. Dis. Commun.* **4**, 57–63.

TREVARTHEN, C. and MARWICK, H. (1986). Signs of motivation for speech in infants and the nature of a mother's support for development of language. In: *Precursors of Early*

Speech, B. Lindblom and R. Zetterstrom (Eds). *Werner-Gren International Symposium Series 44.* Basingstoke: Macmillan Press. (New York: Stockton Press.)

TREVARTHEN, C., MURRAY, L. and HUBLEY, P. (1981). Psychology of infants. In: *Scientific Foundations of Paediatrics*, 2nd edn. J. Davis and J. Dobbing (Eds). London: William Heineman Medical.

TUOMI, S.K. and IVANOFF, P. (1977). Incidence of speech and hearing disorders among kindergarten and Grade one children. *Special Educ. Canada.* **51**, 5–8.

TURTON, L.J. (1983). Curriculum concepts for language treatment of children. In: *Treating Language Disorders*, H. Winitz (Ed.). Baltimore: Baltimore University Park Press.

UNITED STATES OF AMERICA PUBLIC LAW (1975). Education for all Handicapped Children Act, PL 94-142.

UNITED STATES OF AMERICA PUBLIC LAW (1986). Education of the Handicapped Act. Amendment Title 1. Handicapped Infants and Toddlers, PL 99-457.

VAN DER LELY, H. and DEWART, H. (1986). Sentence comprehension strategies in specifically language-impaired children. *Br. J. Dis. Commun.* **21**, 291–306.

VAN DER STELT, J.M. and KOOPMANS VAN BEINUM, F.J. (1986). The onset of babbling related to gross motor development. In: *Precursors of Early Speech*, B. Lindblom and R. Zetterstrom (Eds)., *Werner-Gren International Symposium Series 44.* Basingstoke: Macmillan Press. (New York: Stockton Press.)

VAN KLEEK, A. (1981). Children's development of metalinguistic skills. *Communicative Disorders, Vol. 6. 9, An audio journal for continuing education,* New York: Grune & Stratton.

VAN KLEEK, A. (1984). Assessment and intervention: Does 'Meta' matter? In: *Language Learning Disabilities in School Age Children*, G.P. Wallach and K.G. Butler (Eds). Baltimore: Williams & Wilkins.

VENTRY, I. (1980). Effects of hearing loss. Fact or fiction? *J. Speech Hear. Dis.* **45**, 143–156.

WALLACE, M. (1986). *The Silent Twins.* London: Prentice-Hall.

WALTON, J.N., ELLIS, E. and COURT, S.D.M. (1962). Clumsy Children: developmental apraxia and agnosia. *Brain* **85**, 603–612.

WARD, S. (1984). Detecting abnormal auditory behaviours in infancy: the relationship between such behaviours and linguistic development. *Br. J. Dis. Commun.* **19**, 237–251.

WARD, S. and KELLETT, B. (1982). Language disorder resolved? *Br. J. Dis. Commun.* **17**, 32–52.

WARD, S. and MCCARTNEY, E. (1978). Congenital auditory imperception. A follow-up study. *Br. J. Dis. Commun.* **13**, 1–6.

WARNER, J.A.W. (1987). Cerebral palsy: a chance to influence the environment. *Speech Ther. Pract.* **2**, 5–7.

WARNER, J., BYERS-BROWN, B. and MCCARTNEY, E. (1984). *Speech Therapy: A Clinical Companion.* Manchester: Manchester University Press.

WEDELL, K. (1980). Early Intervention. In: *Early Identification and Treatment of Hyperactive Children*, R.N. Knight and D.J. Bakker (Eds). Baltimore: University Park Press.

WEEKS, T. (1974). *The Slow Speech Development of a Bright Child.* Mass: Lexington Books.

WEINER, P. and HOOCK, W. (1973). The standardization of tests: criteria and criticisms. *J. Speech Hear. Res.* **16**, 616–626.

WEISTUCH, L. and BYERS BROWN, B. (1987). Motherese as therapy: programme and its dissemination. *Child Lang. Teach. Ther.* **3**, 57–72.

WELLS, G. (1985). *Language Development in the Pre-school Years.* Cambridge: Cambridge University Press.

WEST, P. (1969). *Words for a Deaf Daughter.* London: Victor Gollancz.

WETHERBY, A., CAIN, D., YONELAS, A. and WALKER, V. (1986). Intentional communication in the emerging language of normal infants. Mini-seminar presentation at Annual Convention of American Speech, Language and Hearing Association, Detroit.

WHITEHURST, G.J., FALCO, F.L., LONIGEN, C.J., FISCHEL, J.E., DE BARYSHE, B.D., VALDEZ-MANCHAEA, MC. and CAULFIELD, M. (1988). Accelerating language development through picture book reading. *Dev. Psychol.* 24, 690–699.

WICKELGREN, W.A. (1969). Context-sensitive coding, associative memory and serial coding in (speech) behavior. *Psychol. Rev.* 76, 1–15.

WICKELGREN, W.A. (1979). *Cognitive Psychology.* Englewood Cliffs, NJ: Prentice Hall.

WIIG, E. (1987). Strategic language use in adolescents with learning disabilities: Assessment and education. *Proceedings of First International Symposium: Specific Speech and Language Disorders in Children*, University of Reading. London: AFASIC.

WIIG, E. and BECKER-CAPLAN, L. (1984). Linguistic retrieval strategies and word-finding difficulties among children with language disabilities. *Topics Lang. Dis.* 4, 1–18.

WIIG, E. and SEMEL, E. (1976). *Language Disabilities in Children and Adolescents.* Columbus, Ohio: Charles E. Merrill.

WIIG, E. and SEMEL, E. (1980). *Language Assessment and Intervention for the Learning-disordered.* Columbus, Ohio: Charles E. Merrill.

WIIG, E. and SEMEL, E. (1984). *Learning Assessment and Intervention for the Learning Disabled.* Columbus, Ohio: Charles E. Merrill.

WILLIAMS, R., INGHAM, R. and ROSENTHAL, J. (1981). A further analysis for developmental apraxia of speech in children with defective articulation. *J. Speech Hear. Res.* 24, 496–505.

WILSON, B.C (1979). Precursors of learning disabilities. Paper presented at the International Neuropsychological Society, Noordurjerhoot, The Netherlands.

WILSON, B.C. (1981). Longitudinal studies of preschool language-disordered children. Paper presented at The Orton Society Conference, New York.

WILSON, B.C. and RISUCCI, D.A. (1986). A model for clinical quantitative classification: Generation 1. Application to language-disordered pre-school children. *Brain Lang.* 27, 281–309.

WINITZ, H. (1969). *Articulatory Acquisition and Behavior.* New York: Appleton-Century-Crofts.

WOLFF, P.H., GUNNOE, C. and COHEN, C. (1985). Neuromotor maturation and psychological performance: a developmental study. *Dev. Med Child Neurol.* 27, 344–354.

WOLFUS B., MOSCOVITCH, M. and KINSBOURNE, M. (1980). Subgroups of developmental language impairment. *Brain Lang.* 10, 152–171.

WOODS, B.T. and CAREY, S. (1979). Language deficits after apparent recovery from childhood aphasia. Ann. Neurol. 6, 405–409.

WORLD HEALTH ORGANISATION (1980). *Early Detection of Handicap in Children.* Geneva: WHO.

WORSTER-DROUGHT, C. (1965). Observations of congenital auditory imperception. *The Teacher of the Deaf.*

WORSTER-DROUGHT, C. and ALLEN, I.M. (1930). Congenital auditory imperception. *J. Neurol. Psychopathol.* 10, 193–236.

WRIGHT, N.E., THISTLETHWAITE, D., ELTON, R.A., WILKINSON, E.M. and FORFAR, J.O. (1983). The speech and language development of low birthweight infants. *Br. J. Dis. Commun.* 18, 187–196.

YOSS, K.A. and DARLEY, F.L. (1974a). Developmental apraxia of speech in children with defective articulation. *J. Speech Hear. Res.* 17, 399–416.

YOSS, K.A. and DARLEY, F.L. (1974b). Therapy in developmental apraxia of speech. *Lang. Speech Hear. Services in Schools* 5, 23–31.

Principal Tests cited in Text

ANTHONY, A., BOGLE, D., INGRAM, T.T.S. and MCISAAC, M. (1971). *Edinburgh Articulation Test*. Edinburgh: Livingstone.

ARTHUR, G. (1952). *Leiter International Performance Scale* (adaptation). Washington DC: Psychological Services Center.

BAYLEY, N. (1969). *Bayley Scales of Infant Development*. New York: Psychological Corp.

BISHOP, D.V.M. (1983). *Test for Reception of Grammar*. Available from the author, Dept of Psychology, University of Manchester.

CAPUTE, A.J., PALMER, F.B., SHAPIRO, B.K., WACHTEL, R.C., SCHMIDT, S. and ROSS, A. (1986). Clinical and Auditory Milestone Scale. Prediction of cognition in infancy. *Dev. Med. Child Neurol.* **28**, 762–771.

CARROW WOLFOLK, E. (1973, revised 1985). *Test for Auditory Comprehension of Language*. Windsor: NFER.

CARROW WOLFOLK, E. (1974). *Carrow Elicited Language Inventory*. Windsor: NFER.

DEWART, H. and SUMMERS, S. (1988). *Pragmatic and Early Communication Profile*. Windsor: NFER.

DOLL, E.A. (1965). *Vineland Maturity Scale*. Minneapolis: American Guidance Service.

FRANKENBURG, W.K., FANDAL, A.W., SCIARELTO, W. and BURGESS, D. (1981). The Newly Abbreviated and Revised Denver Developmental Screening Test. *J. Pediatr.* **99**, 995–999.

FRENCH, J.L. (1964). *Pictorial Test of Intelligence*. New York: Houghton Mifflin.

GOLDMAN, R., FRISTOE, N. and WOODCOCK, R.W. (1972). *Goldman–Fristoe–Woodcock Test of Auditory Discrimination*. Circle Pines, Minneapolis: American Guidance Service.

GRUNWELL, P. (1982). *Phonological Assessment of Children's Speech*. Windsor: NFER.

GUTFREUND, M. (1988). *Bristol Language Development Scales*. Windsor: NFER.

HEDRICK, D.L., PRATHER, E.M. and TOBIN, A.E. (1975). *Sequenced Inventory of Communication Development*. Seattle: Seattle University Press.

HISKEY, M.S. (1966). *Hiskey–Nebraska Test of Learning Aptitude*. Lincoln: Union College Press.

KIRK, S.A., MCCARTHY, J.J. and KIRK, W.D. (1968). *Illinois Test of Psycholinguistic Abilities*. Urbana, Ill: University of Illinois Press.

KOIKE, K.J.M. and ASP, C.W. (1981). Tennessee Test of Rhythm and Intonation Patterns (T-TRIP). *J. Speech Hear. Dis.* **46**, 81–87.

LEE, L. (1969). *North Western Syntax Screening Test*. Evanstown: North Western University Press.

MCCARTHY, D. (1974). *McCarthy Scales of Children's Abilities.* New York: Psychological Corp.

MEECHAM, N. (1958). *Verbal Language Development Scale,* Revised, 1971. Circle Pines, MN: American Guidance Service.

MORGAN-BARRIE, P. (1988). *Auditory Discrimination and Attention Test.* Windsor: NFER.

RENFREW, C.E. (1972). Auditory Discrimination Test. Obtainable from the author, 2a North Place, Old Headington, Oxford OX3 9HX.

RENFREW, C.E. (1972). The Bus Story. Obtainable from author – see above.

RENFREW, C.E. (1988). Action Picture Test (revised). Obtainable from the author – see above.

REYNELL, J. (1977; 1985 revised edn). *Reynell Language Development Scales.* Windsor: NFER.

TEMPLIN, M. (1957). *Certain Language Skills in Children.* Minneapolis: University of Minnesota Press.

WECHSLER, D. (1967). *Wechsler Pre-school and Primary Scale of Intelligence (WIPPSI).* New York: Psychological Corp.

WEINER, F.F. (1979). *Natural Process Analysis.* Baltimore: University Park Press.

WEPMAN, J. (1973). *Auditory Discrimination Test.* Chicago: Language Research Association.

WIIG, E.H. (1982). *Clinical Evaluation of Language Functions: CELF-R.* Sidcup: Kent Psychological Corp.

Glossary

Allophone A phonetic realisation. The manner in which a phoneme varies subject to the influence of, for example, adjacent phones

Anarthria Complete inability to articulate sounds. Both voice and resonance are affected. Neuropathological in origin. **Dysarthria** is a less severe form.

Angular gyrus The posterior part of the parietal lobe of the brain concerned with the integration of sensory input.

Arcuate fasciculus Neural pathway connecting Wernicke's (temporal) and Broca's (anterior motor) areas of cerebral cortex.

Basal ganglia Collection of subcortical neuronal areas. Through their connection with the cerebral cortex and the cerebellum they influence rate and accuracy of movement. As part of the limbic system they also function as regulators of emotion.

Brain stem Serves as a connection between cerebrum and spinal cord. Comprises mid-brain, pons and medulla oblongata. Regulates many vital functions including respiration and the cardiovascular system.

Broca's area Anterior area of the cerebral cortex concerned with the planning and organisation of speech.

Cerebellum Part of the brain which regulates and modifies movement through input from sensory pathways and through its connections with subcortical and cortical areas.

Diadochokinesis In speech, is the inability to carry out rapid alternating and repetitive movements of the articulatory organs.

Dopamine A neurotransmitter originating in the cells of the substantia nigra and corpus striatum (basal ganglia). Deficiencies lead to severe motor disorders, e.g. Parkinson's disease.

Dysarthria See Anarthria.

Gilles de la Tourette syndrome A neurological condition characterised by involuntary tics, both facial and vocal, expiratory noises, echolalia.

Haptic perception That which derives from tactile and proprioceptive input.

Heschls gyrus   A transverse convolution in the dominant temporal lobe particularly concerned with synthesis of incoming auditory signals.

Hippocampus   Part of the limbic system involved in the retention of short-term episodic memory possibly through its influence on cortical cells.

Hyperlexia   Abnormally advanced reading ability without necessarily understanding the content.

Illocution   A term used in speech act theory; that which involves the speaker directly, e.g. thanking, promising, describing. Compare **perlocution** where the speaker's utterance has an effect upon the listener. Note: Piagetian theory uses this term to denote action accompanying verbalisation.

Lexicon   The store of linguistic knowledge concerning structural properties of a language.

Logogens   Lexical stores. A logogen collects information relating to the word it stores via perceptual pathways. It is connected both to the semantic/cognitive system enabling meaning to be accessed and to the response system so that the appropriate word may be produced (Logogen theory proposed by Morton, 1968, 1978).

Medial geniculate body   A nucleus on the posterior surface of the thalamus. It receives information from the organ of Corti of the contralateral ear. It is concerned with differentiation of pitch. Its fibres terminate in the auditory region of the temporal lobe.

Metalinguistics   The study of awareness of the properties of language.

Metathesis   In linguistics, a change in the sequence of sounds, syllables or words within an utterance, e.g. spoonerisms.

Morpheme   The smallest functional unit of language relating to the composition of words.

Myelin   A protective covering for the nerve fibres. Its presence facilitates speed of transmission. Myelination of certain nerve pathways is a maturational feature.

Organ of Corti   A sensory part of the cochlea of the ear. The function of its receptors is to convert sound pressure waves into electrical impulses which are transmitted via the eighth cranial nerve to the brain. See Medial geniculate body.

Paradigmatic response   In psycholinguistics, a term used to describe associated responses to a stimulus word. Paradigmatic responses are in the same word class, e.g. cake–bread–biscuit. Compare Syntagmatic.

Phonology   The study of contrastive sound systems within a specific language.

Pragmatics   A linguistic term which describes the study of the way in which language is used in social interaction.

Proprioception   Awareness of movements of the body, in this context with special reference to movements within the vocal tract (also Kinaesthesia).

Prosody   The melody of a language determined by non-segmental features of pitch, stress, loudness and timing.

Pyramidal cells   Large nerve cells found predominantly in the motor cortex of the brain, also to some extent in somaesthetic areas. They give rise to the pyramidal tract crucially concerned in initiation of motor activity.

Reticular system   A network of nuclei and fibres within the medulla oblongata. One of its functions is to maintain appropriate levels of muscular tension throughout the body including the vocal tract.

Semantics   The study of the meaning of language.

Supplementary motor cortex   An area on the medial surface of the cerebral hemisphere adjacent to the motor and somaesthetic strips. Its function may be concerned with the timing and sequential aspects of speech production.

Syntagmatic   In psycholinguistics an associated response involving a different word category, e.g. bed–sleep–dream.

Syntax   The study of the way in which words relate to one another in a language.

Taxonomy   Classification and categorisation, e.g. parts of speech.

Thalamus   A collection of nuclei situated subcortically. Its functions in many respects mirror those of the cerebral cortex. An important way station for both motor and sensory pathways. It is also involved in affective aspects of speech.

Tone   The syllable within a tone on which a change of pitch occurs.

Tone group   A stretch of speech extending from six to eight syllables having one prominant tone, the nuclear stress.

Tonicity   The syllable within a tone unit which carries maximum stress.

Visispeech   Instrumentation which records and displays on a screen, intonation and stress patterns generated by a speaker.

Vocable   Babble used meaningfully.

Wernicke's area   Region in the superior part of the temporal lobe of the cerebral cortex. Its function relates to the understanding of spoken language.

Author Index

Subject Index

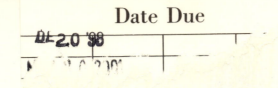

Date Due

DEC 20 '98